General Knowledge

Compiled & Edited
Research & Editorial Deptt.

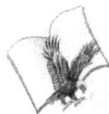

V&S PUBLISHERS

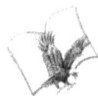

Published by:

V&S PUBLISHERS

F-2/16, Ansari road, Daryaganj, New Delhi-110002
☎ 23240026, 23240027 • *Fax:* 011-23240028
Email: info@vspublishers.com • *Website:* www.vspublishers.com

Regional Office : Hyderabad
5-1-707/1, Brij Bhawan (Beside Central Bank of India Lane)
Bank Street, Koti, Hyderabad - 500 095
☎ 040-24737290
E-mail: vspublishershyd@gmail.com

Branch Office : Mumbai
Jaywant Industrial Estate, 1st Floor–108, Tardeo Road
Opposite Sobo Central Mall, Mumbai – 400 034
☎ 022-23510736
E-mail: vspublishersmum@gmail.com

Follow us on: 🇹 f in

Printed at Repro Knowledgecast Limited, Thane

PUBLISHER'S NOTE

V&S Publishers is constant in its effort to identify the problems faced by the aspirants of various competitive examinations held at state and national levels, and to sort out those problems effectively. After a thorough search in the market, we realised that there are a few books available on comprehensive General Knowledge, which are too costly and too large to go through in short span of time during preparation. The present book, **'General Knowledge'** with all genres of general awareness has been designed to meet the specific needs of the contestants of various entrance exams and competitive exams as well. Not only does the book spreads awareness, but also can be a facilitator of change in life.

The book has been strategically planned in order to be user friendly. It covers up-to-date knowledge on *Physics, Chemistry, Biology & Computers*. The primary goal is to fulfil the quest for knowledge on various topics of study at national and international levels.

The book is recommended for various competitive examinations such as:

⇨ Civil Services
⇨ Staff Selection Commission (SSC)
⇨ Institute of Banking Personnel Selection (IBPS)
⇨ Defence Services – CDSE, NDA and other defence services
⇨ Management Aptitude Test (MAT), Common Admission Test (CAT), and Graduate Management Admission Test (GMAT)
⇨ Indian Engineering Services
⇨ Railway Recruitment Services
⇨ Test of English as a Foreign Language (TOEFL)
⇨ International English Language Testing System (IELTS)

We hope that the book will be of immense help to the readers to up-grade their knowledge on various topics of general knowledge. A regular revision of all the topics covered in the book is advised to get up-to-date with the required information. We wish all aspirants good luck for their future endeavours.

CONTENTS

GENERAL SCIENCE

Physics

1. Unit

Unit : The chosen standard used for measuring a physical quantity is called unit.

Unit should be :

(i) well defined   (ii) easy to reproduce

(iii) easy to compare   (v) internationally accepted

(iv) independent of changes in physical conditions

Units are of two types– (i) Fundamental unit; (i) Derived unit

System of Units– Units depend on choice. Each choice of units leads to a new system (set) of units. The internationally accepted systems are (i) CGS system, (ii) MKS system (iii) FPS system (iv) SI units.

In SI Units, there are seven fundamental units given in the following table:

Physical Quantity	SI Unit	Symbol	Physical Quantity	SI Unit	Symbol
Length	metre	m	Temperature	kelvin	K
Mass	kilogram	kg	Luminuous intensity	candela	Cd
Time	second	s	Amount of substance	mole	mol
Electric Current	ampere	A			

Besides these seven fundamental units, two supplementary units are also defined, viz., radian [rad] for plane angle and steradian (sr) for solid angle.

⇨ All the units which are defined/expressed in terms of fundamental units are called derived units.

Some important derived units are:

S. No.	Physical Quantity	CGS units	SI unit	Relation
1.	Force	dyne	newton	1 newton = 10^5 dyne
2.	work	erg	joule	1 joule = 10^7 erg

Some practical units of length, mass and time

Length	Mass	Time
Light year = distance travelled by light in one year in vaccum.	1 quintal = 10^2 kg	1 solar day = 86400 sec.
1 ly = 9.46×10^{15} cm	1 metric ton = 10^3 kg	1 year = 365 solar days
1 astronomical unit (A.U.)	1 atomic mass unit (amu)	1 lunar month
$\quad$ = 1.5×10^{11} m	or dalton = 1.66×10^{-27} kg	$\quad$ = 27.3 solar days.
1 parsec = 3.26 ly	1 slug = 1459 kg	**Tropical year** = It is the year in which total solar eclipse occurs.
$\quad$ = 3.08×10^{16} m	1 pound = 0.4537 kg	
1 nautical mile or seamile	1 Chandrashekhar	**Leap year** = It is the year in which the month of February is of 29 days.
$\quad$ = 6020 ft.	limit =	
1 micron= 1 μm =10^{-6} m	1.4 times the mass of	
1 angstron (A°) = 10^{-15} m	sun = 2.8×10^{30} kg	

Prefixes used in metric system

Prefix	Symbol	Multiplier	Prefix	Symbol	Multiplier
deci	d	10^{-1}	deca	da	10^{1}
centi	c	10^{-2}	hecto	n	10^{2}
milli	m	10^{-3}	kilo	k	10^{3}
micro	μ	10^{-6}	mega	M	10^{6}
nano	n	10^{-9}	giga	G	10^{9}
pico	n	10^{-12}	tera	T	10^{12}
femto	f	10^{-15}	peta	P	10^{15}
atto	a	10^{-18}	exa	E	10^{18}
zepto	z	10^{-21}	zetta	Z	10^{21}
yocto	y	10^{-24}	yotta	Y	10^{24}

2. Motion

Scalar Quantities : Physical quantities which have magnitude only and no direction are called *scalar quantities*.

Example : Mass, speed, volume, work, time, power, energy etc.

Vector Quantities : Physical quantities which have magnitude and direction both and which obey triangle law are called *vector quantities*.

Example : Displacement, velocity, acceleration, force, momentum, torque etc.

Electric current, though has a direction, is a scalar quantity because it does not obey triangle law.

Moment of inertia, pressure, refractive index, stress are tensor quantities.

Distance : Distance is the length of actual path covered by a moving object in a given time interval.

Displacement: Shortest distance covered by a body in a definite direction is called *displacement*.

⇨ Distance is a scalar quantity whereas displacement is a vector quantity both having the same unit (metre).

⇨ Displacement may be positive, negative or zero whereas distance is always positive.

⇨ In general, magnitude of displacement ≤ distance

Speed : Distance travelled by the moving object in unit time interval is called speed i.e. speed = Distance/Time

It is a scalar quantity and its SI unit is metre/second (m/s).

Velocity : Velocity of a moving object is defined as the displacement of the object in unit time interval i.e. velocity = Displacement/Time

It is a vector quantity and its SI unit is metre/second.

Acceleration : Acceleration of an object is defined as the rate of change of velocity of the object i.e. acceleration = Change in Velocity/Time

It is a vector quantity and its SI units is metre/second^2 (m/s^2)

If velocity decreases with time then acceleration is negative and is called retardation.

Circular Motion : It an object describes a circular path (circle) its motion is called circular motion. If the object moves with uniform speed, its motion is uniform circular motion.

Uniform circular motion is an accelerated motion because the direction of velocity changes continuously.

Angular Velocity : The angle subtended by the line joining the object from the origin of circle in unit time interval is called angular velocity.

It is generally denoted by ω and $\omega = \theta/t$

If T = time period = time taken by the object to complete one revolution, n = frequency = no. of revolutions in one second.

then $\boxed{nT = 1}$ & $\omega = 2\pi/T = 2\pi n$

⇨ In one revolution, the object travels $2\pi r$ distance.

Linear speed = ωr = angular speed × radius

Newton's laws of motion: Newton, the father of physics established the laws of motion in his book "principia" in 1667.

Newton's first law of motion: Every body maintains its initial state of rest or motion with uniform speed on a straight line unless an external force acts on it.

⇨ First law is also called law of *Galileo* or *law of inertia*.

⇨ **Inertia:** Inertia is the property of a body by virtue of which the body opposes change in its initial state of rest or motion with uniform speed on a straight line.

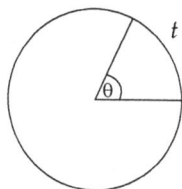

Inertia is of two types (i) Inertia of rest (ii) Inertia of motion

Some examples of Inertia :

(i) When a car or train starts suddenly, the passengers bends backward.

(ii) When a running horse stops suddenly, the rider bends forward.

(iii) When a coat/blanket is beaten by a stick, the dust particles are removed.

⇨ First law gives the definition of force.

⇨ **Force :** Force is that external cause which when acts on a body changes or tries to change the initial state of the body.

Momentum : Momentum is the property of a moving body and is defined as the product of mass and velocity of the body i.e.

momentum = mass × velocity.

It is a vector quantity. Its SI unit is kgm/s.

Newton's second law of motion: The rate of change in momentum of a body is directly proportional to the applied force on the body and takes place in the direction of force:

If F = force applied, a = acceleration produced and

m = mass of body the $nF = ma$.

⇨ Newton's second law gives the magnitude of force.

⇨ Newton's first law is contained in the second law.

Newton's Third Law of Motion: To every action, there is an equal and opposite reaction.

Examples of third law-(i) Recoil of a gun (ii) Motion of rocket (iii) Swimming (iv) While drawing water from the well, if the string breaks up the man drawing water falls back.

Principle of conservation of linear momentum : If no external force acts on a system of bodies, the total linear momentum of the system of bodies remains constant.

As a consequence, the total momentum of bodies before and after collision remains the same.

Impulse : When a large force acts on a body for very small time, then force is called impulsive force. Impulse is defined as the product of force and time.

Impulse = force × time = change in momentum.

⇨ It is a vector quantity and its direction is the direction of force. Its SI unit is newton second (Ns).

Centripetal Force: When a body travels along a circular path, its velocity changes continuously. Naturally an external force always acts on the body towards the centre of the path.

The external force required to maintain the circular motion of the body is called *centripetal force.*

If a body of mass m is moving on a circular path of radius R with uniform speed v, then the required centripetal force, $F = mv^2/R$

Centrifugal Force: In applying the Newton's laws of motion, we have to consider some forces which can not be assigned to any object in the surrounding. These forces are called pseudo force or inertial force.

Centrifugal force is such a pseudo force. It is equal and opposite to centripetal force.

⇨ Cream separator, centrifugal drier work on the principle of centrifugal force.

⇨ Centrifugal force should not be confused as the reaction to centripetal force because *forces of action and reaction act on different bodies.*

Moment of force : The rotational effect of a force on a body about an axis of rotation is described in terms of moment of force.

Moment of a force about an axis of rotation is measured as the product of magnitude of force and the perpendicular distance of direction of force from the axis of rotation.

i.e., Moment of force = Force × moment arm

⇨ It is a vector quantity.

⇨ Its SI unit is newton metre (Nm)

Centre of Gravity : The centre of gravity of a body is that point through which the entire weight of body acts. The centre of gravity of a body does not change with the change in orientation of body in space.

The weight of a body acts through centre of gravity in the downward direction. Hence a body can be brought to equilibrium by applying a force equal to its weight in the vertically upward direction through centre of gravity.

Equilibrium : If the resultant of all the forces acting on a body is zero then the body is said to be in equilibrium.

If a body is in equilibrium, it will be either at rest or in uniform motion.

If it is at rest, the equilibrium is called static, otherwise dynamic.

Static equilibrium is of the following three types :

(i) Stable Equilibrium : If on slight displacement from equilibrium position, a body has tendency to regain its original position, it is said to be in stable equilibrium.

(ii) Unstable Equilibrium : If on slight displacement from equilibrium position, a body moves in the direction of displacement and does not regain its original position, the equilibrium is said to unstable equilibrium . In this equilibrium, the centre of gravity of the body is at the highest position.

(iii) Neutral Equilibrium : If on slight displacement from equilibrium position a body has no tendency to come back to its original position or to move in the direction of displacement, it is said to be in neutral equilibrium. In neutral equilibrium, the centre of gravity always remains at the same height.

Conditions for Stable Equilibrium : For stable equilibrium of a body, the following two conditions should be fulfilled.

(i)   The centre of gravity of the body should be at the minimum height.

(ii) The vertical line passing through the centre of gravity of the body should pass through the base of the body.

3. Work, Energy and Power

Work : If a body gets displaced when a force acts on it, work is said to be done. Work is measured by the product of force and displacement of the body along the direction of force.

If a body gets displaced by S when a force F acts on it,

then the work $W = F\,S\,\cos\theta$

where θ = angle between force and displacement

If both force and displacement are in the same direction, then $W = FS$

Work is a scalar quantity and its SI unit is joule.

Energy : Capacity of doing work by a body is called its energy.

⇨   Energy is a scalar quantity and its SI unit is joule.

⇨   Energy developed in a body due to work done on it is called mechanical energy. Mechanical energy is of two types :

(i) Potential Energy (ii) Kinetic Energy

Potential Energy : The capacity of doing work developed in a body due to its position or configuration is called its potential energy.

Example : (i) energy of stretched or compressed spring (ii) energy of water collected at a height (iii) energy of spring in a watch.

PE of a body in the gravitational field of earth is *mgh*.

where *m* = mass, *g* = acceleration due to gravity, *h* = height of the body from surface of the earth.

Kinetic Energy : Energy possess by a body due to its motion is called Kinetic Energy of the body.

If a body of mass *m* is moving with speed v, then kinetic energy of the body is $\dfrac{1}{2}\,mv^{2}$

Principle of Conservation of Energy

Energy can neither be created nor can be destroyed. Only energy can be transformed from one form to another form. Whenever energy is utilized in one form, equal amount of energy is produced in other form. Hence total energy of the universe always remains the same. This is called the principle of conservation of energy.

Some Equipments used to Transform Energy

S. No.	Equipment	Energy Transformed
1.	Dynamo	Mechanical energy into electrical energy
2.	Candle	Chemical energy into light and heat energy.
3.	Microphone	Sound energy into electrical energy.
4.	Loud speaker	Electrical energy into sound energy.
5.	Solar cell	Solar energy into electrical energy.
6.	Tube light	Electrical energy into light energy.
7.	Electric bulb	Electrical energy into light and heat energy.
8.	Battery	Chemical energy into electrical energy.
9.	Electric motor	Electrical energy into mechanical energy.
10.	Sitar	Mechanical energy into sound energy.

Relation between Momentum and Kinetic Energy

$$\text{K.E.} = \frac{p^2}{2m} \text{ where } p = \text{momentum} = mv$$

Clearly when momentum is doubled, kinetic energy becomes four times.

Power : Rate of doing work is called power.

⇨ It an agent does W work in time t, then power of agent $= \dfrac{W}{t}$

SI unit of power is watt named as a respect to the scientist James Watt.

watt = joule/sec.

1 kW = 10^3 watt

1 MW = 10^6 watt

Horse power is a practical unit of power. 1 H.P. = 746 watt.

1 watt second = 1 watt × 1 second = 1 joule.

1 watt hour (Wh) = 3600 joule

1 kilowatt hour (kWh) = 3.6×10^6 joule.

W, kW, MW & H.P. are units of power.

Ws, Wh, kWh are units of work and energy.

4. Gravitation

Gravitation : Every body attracts other body by a force called force of gravitation.

Newton's law of Gravitation : The force of gravitational attraction between two point bodies is directly proportional to the product of their masses and inversely proportional to the square of the distance between them.

Consider two point bodies of masses m_1 and m_2 are plaqed at a distance r. The force of gravitational attraction between them, $F = G\dfrac{m_1 m_2}{r^2}$

Here G is constant called universal gravitational constant. The value of G is 6.67×10^{-11} Nm^2/kg^2.

Gravity : The gravitational force of earth is called gravity i.e. gravity is the force by which earth pulls a body towards its centre.

The acceleration produced in a body due to force of gravity is called acceleration due to gravity (denoted as g) and its value is 9.8 m/s^2

⇨ Acceleration due to gravity is independent of shape, size and mass of the body.

Variation in g

(i) value of g decreases with height or depth from earth's surface.

(ii) g is maximum at poles.

(iii) g is minimum at equator.

(iv) g decreases due to rotation of earth.

(v) g decreases if angular speed of earth increases and increases if angular speed of earth decreases.

⇨ If angular speed of earth becomes 17 times its present value, a body on the equator becomes weightless.

Weight of a body in a lift

(i) If lift is stationary or moving with uniform speed (either upward or down ward), the apparent weight of a body is equal to its true weight.

(ii) If lift is going up with acceleration, the apparent weight of a body is more than the true weight.

(iii) If lift is going down with acceleration, the apparent weight of a body is less than the true weight.

(iv) If the cord of the lift is broken, it falls freely. In this situation the weight of a body in the lift becomes zero. This is the situation of weight lessness.

(v) While going down, if the acceleration of lift is more than acceleration due to gravity, a body in the lift goes in contact of the ceiling of lift.

Kepler's Laws of planetary motion

(i) All planets move around the sun in elliptical orbits, with the sun being at rest at one focus of the orbit.

(ii) The position vector of the planet with sun at the origin sweeps out equal area in equal time i.e. The areal yelocity of planet around the sun always remains constant.

A consequence of this law is that the speed of planet increases when the planet is closer to the sun and decreases when the planet is far away from sun.

Speed of a planet is maximum when it is at perigee and minimum when it is at apogee.

(iii) The square of the period of revolution of a planet around the sun is directly proportional to the cube of mean distance of planet from the sun.

If T is period of revolution and r is the mean distance of planet from sun then $T^2 \propto r^3$.

Clearly distant planets have larger period of revolution. The time period of nearest planet Mercury is 88 days where as time period of farthest planet Pluto is 247.7 years.

Satellite : Satellites are natural or artificial bodies revolving around a planet under its gravitational attraction. Moon is a natural satellite while INSAT-IB is an artificial satellite of earth.

Orbital speed of a satellite

(i) Orbital speed of a satellite is independent of its mass. Hence satellites of different masses revolving in the orbit of same radius have same orbital speed.

(ii) Orbital speed of a satellite depends upon the radius of orbit (height of satellite from the surface of earth). Greater the radius of orbit, lesser will be the orbital speed.

⇨ The orbital speed of a satellite revolving near the surface of earth is 7.9 km/sec.

Period of Revolution of a satellite : Time taken by a satellite to complete one revolution in its orbit is called its period of revolution.

i.e. period of revolution = $\dfrac{\text{circumference of orbit}}{\text{orbital speed}}$

(i) Period of revolution of a satellite depends upon the height of satellite from the surface of earth. Greater the height, more will be the period of revolution.

(ii) Period of revolution of a satellite is independent of its mass.

⇨ The period of revolution of satellite revolving near the surface of earth is 1 hour 24 minute (84 minute)

Geo-Stationary Satellite : If a satellite revolves in equatorial plane in the direction of earth's rotation i.e. from west to east with a period of revolution equal to time period of rotation of earth on its own axis i.e. 24 hours, then the satellite will appear stationary relative to earth. Such a satellite is called Geo-*stationary satellite.* Such a satellite revolves around the earth at a height of 36000 km. The orbit of Geo stationary satellite is called *parking orbit. Arthur C. Clarck* was first to predict that a communication satellite can be stationed in the geo synchronous orbit.

Escape velocity : Escape velocity is that minimum velocity with which a body should be projected from the surface of earth so as it goes out of gravitational field of earth and never return to earth.

⇨ Escape velocity is independent of the mass, shape and size of the body and its direction of projection.
⇨ Escape velocity is also called second cosmic velocity.
⇨ For earth, escape velocity= 11.2 km/s.
For moon, escape velocity= 2.4 km/s.

Orbital velocity of a satellite $V_0 = \sqrt{g}\ R$ and escape velocity $V_e = \sqrt{2gR}$

where R = Radius of earth i.e. $V_e = \sqrt{2}\ V_0$ i.e. escape velocity is √2. times the orbital velocity.

Therefore if the orbital velocity of a satellite is increased to √2 times (increased by 41%), the satellite will leave the orbit and escape.

5. Pressure

Pressure : Pressure is defined as force acting normally on unit area of the surface.

$$\text{Pressure (P)} = \frac{F}{A} = \frac{\text{Normal force on the surface}}{\text{Area of the surface}}$$

SI unit of pressure is N/m^2 also called pascal (Pa). Pressure is a scalar quantity.

Atmospheric Pressure : Atmospheric pressure is that pressure which is exerted by a mercury column of 76 cm length at 0°C at 45° latitude at the sea-level. It is equal to weight of 76 cm column of mercury of cross sectional area 1 cm². Generally it is measured in bar. 1 bar = $10^5\ N/m^2$

Atmospheric pressure 1 atm = 1.01 bar = $1.01 \times 10^5\ N/m^2$ = 760 torr
⇨ One torr is the pressure exerted by a mercury column of 1mm length.
⇨ Atmospheric pressure decreases with altitude (height from earth's surface). This is why (i) It is difficult to cook on the mountain (ii) The fountain pen of a passenger leaks in aeroplane at height.
⇨ Atmospheric pressure is measured by barometer. With the help of barometer, weather forecast can be made.
⇨ Sudden fall in barometric reading is the indication of storm.
⇨ Slow fall in barometric reading is the indication of rain.
⇨ Slow rise in the barometric reading is the indication of clear weather.

Pressure in liquid : Force exerted on unit area of wall or base of the container by the molecules of liquid is the pressure of liquid .

The pressure exerted by liquid at depth h below the surface of liquid is given as $p = hdg$ where d is the density of liquid.
⇨ Regarding pressure, the following points are worth noting :
  (i) In a static liquid at same horizontal level, pressure is same at all points.
  (ii) Pressure at a point in a static liquid has same value in all directions.
  (iii) Pressure at a point in a liquid is proportional to the depth of the point from the free surface.

(iv) Pressure at a point in a liquid is proportional to the density of the liquid.

Pascal law for pressure of liquid

(i) If gravitational attraction is negligible, in equilibrium condition, pressure is same at all points in a liquid.

(ii) If an external pressure is applied to an exclosed fluid, it is transmitted undiminished to every direction.

⇨ Hydrolic lift, hydrolic press, Hydrolic brake work on Pascal law.

Effect of pressure on Melting Point and Boiling Point

(i) The M.P. of substances which expands on fusion increases with the increase in pressure; for example - wax.

(ii) The M.P. of substances which contracts on fusion decreases with the increase in temperature for example - ice.

(iii) Boiling point of all the substances increases with the increase in pressure.

6. Floatation

Buoyant Force : When a body is immersed party or wholly in a liquid, a force acts on the body by the liquid in the upward direction. This force is called Buoyant force or force of buoyancy or upthrust. It is equal to the weight of liquid displaced by the body and acts at the centre of gravity of displaced liquid. Its study was first made by Archimedes.

Archimedes Principle : When a body is immersed partly or wholly in a liquid, there is an apparent loss in the weight of the body which is equal to the weight of liquid displaced by the body.

Law of Floatation

A body floats in a liquid if

(i) Density of material of body is less than or equal to the density of liquid.

(ii) If density of material of body is equal to density of liquid, the body floats fully submerged in liquid in neutral equilibrium.

(iii) When body floats in neutral equilibrium, the weight of the body is equal to the weight of displaced liquid.

(iv) The centre of gravity of the body and centre of gravity of the displaced liquid should be in one vertical line.

Centre of Buoyancy : The centre of gravity of the liquid displaced by a body is called centre of buoyancy.

Meta Centre : When a floating body is slightly tilted from equilibrium position, the centre of buoyancy shifts. The point at which the vertical line passing through the new position of centre of buoyancy meets with the initial line is called meta centre.

Conditions for stable equilibrium of Floating body

(i) The meta centre must always be higher than the centre gravity of the body.

(ii) The line joining the centre of gravity of the body and centre of flotation should be vertical.

Density : Density is defined as mass per unit volume.

$$\text{Density} = \frac{\text{mass}}{\text{volume}}. \text{ Its SI unit is kg/m}^3.$$

$$\text{Relative density} = \frac{\text{density of material}}{\text{density of water at } 4°C}$$

Since relative density is a ratio, it is unitless.

⇨ Relative density is measured by Hydrometer .

⇨ The density of sea water is more than that of normal water. This explains why it is easier to swim in sea water.

⇨ When ice floats ih water, its 1/10 the part remain outside the water.

⇨ If ice floating in water in a vessel melts, the level of water in the vessel does not change.

⇨ Purity of milk is measured by lactometer.

7. Surface Tension

Cohesive Force : The force of attraction between the molecules of same substance is called cohesive force. Cohesive force is maximum in solids. This is why solids have a fixed shape. Cohesive force is negligble in case of gases.

Adhesive Force : Force of attraction between the molecules of different substances is called adhesive force. Due to adhesive force, one body sticks to other.

Surface Tension : Surface tension is the property of a liquid by virtue of which it has the tendency to have the area of its free surface minimum as if it were under tension like a stretched elastic membrane.

Surface tension of a liquid is measured by the normal force acting per unit length on either side of an imaginary line drawn on the free surface of liquid and tangential to the free surface.

So, if a force F acts on an imaginary line of length l, then surface tension, $T = F/l$.

⇨ Work done in increasing the surface area of a liquid by unity under isothermal condition is equal to surface tension of liquid. According to this definition, unit of surface tension is joule/meter².

⇨ Surface tension of a liquid decreases with the increase of temperature and becomes zero at critical temperature.

Capillary tube : A tube having very narrow (fine) and uniform bore is called a capillary tube.

Capillarity : If a capillary tube is dipped in a liquid, liquid ascends or descends in the capillary tube. This phenomenon is called capillarity.

⇨ The height by which liquid ascends or decends in a capillary tube depends upon the radius of the tube.

The capillarity depends on the nature of liquid and solid both. The liquid which wets the wall of tube rises in the tube and the liquid which does not wet the wall of tube descends in the tube. For example, when a glass capillary tube is dipped in water, water rises in the tube and shape of water meniscus is concave, similarly when a glass capillary tube is dipped in mercury, mercury decends in the tube and shape of mercury meniscus is convex.

Illustrations of Capillarity

   (i) A piece of blotting paper soaks ink because the pores of the blotting paper serve as capillary tubes,

   (ii) The oil in the wick of a lamp rises due to capillary action of threads in the wick,

   (iii) The root hairs of plants draws water from the soil through capillary action,

   (iv) To prevent loss of water due to capillary action, the soil is loosened and split into pieces by the farmers,

   (v) If a capillary tube is dipped in water in an artificial satellite, water rises up to other end of tube because of its zero apparent weight, how long the tube may be.

   (vi) Action of towel in soaking up water from the body is due to capillary action of cotton in the towel.

   (vii) Melted wax, in a candle rises up to wick by capillary action.

⇨ If a clean and dry needle is very slowly kept on the surface of water, it floats due to surface tension.

⇨ The addition of detergent or soap decrease the surface tension of water and thus increases the cleaning ability.

⇨ Bubbles of soap solution are big because addition of soap decreases the surface tension of water.

⇨ When kerosene oil is sprinkled on water, its surface tension decreases. As a result the larva of mosquitoes floating on the surface of water die due to sinking.

⇨ Warm soup is tasty because at high temperature its surface tension is low and consequently the soup spreads on all parts of the tongue.

8. Viscosity

Visocus Force : The force which opposes the ralative motion between different layers of liquid or gases is called viscous force.

Viscosity : Viscosity is the property of a liquid by virtue of which it opposes the relative motion between its different layers.

⇨ Viscosity is the property of liquids and gases both.

⇨ The viscosity of a liquid is due to cohesive force between its molecules.

⇨ The viscosity of a gas is due to diffusion of its molecules from one layer to other layer.

- Viscosity of gases is much less than that of liquids. There is no viscosity in solids.
- Viscosity of an ideal fluid is zero.
- With rise in temperature, viscosity of liquids decreases and that for gases increases.
- Viscosity of a fluid is measured by its coefficient of viscosity. Its SI unit is decapoise (kg/ms) or pascal second. It is generally denoted by η.

Terminal Velocity : When a body falls in a viscous medium, its velocity first increases and finally becomes constant. This constant velocity is called Terminal velocity.

In this situation, the weight of the body is equal to the sum of viscous force and force of buoyancy i.e. the net force on the body is zero.

Terminal velocity of a spherical body falling in a viscous medium is proportional to the square of radius of the body.

Streamline Flow : If a fluid is flowing in such a way that velocity of all the fluid particles reaching a particular point is same at all time, then the flow of fluid is said to be streamline flow. Thus in streamline flow, each particle follows the same path as followed by a previous particle passing through that point.

Critical Velocity : The maximum velocity up to which fluid motion is streamline is called critical velocity. Clearly, if the velocity of flow is below critical velocity, flow is streamline and of the velocity is above the critical velocity, flow is turbulent.

If the velocity of flow is less than critical velocity, the rate of flow of fluid depends basically on viscosity of fluid. If the velocity of flow is more than critical velocity, the rate of flow deperids on the density of fluid and not on viscosity. Due to this reason, on eruption of the volcano the lava coming out of it flows very swiftly although it is very dense having large viscosity.

Bernoulli's Theorem : According to Bernoulli's theorem, in case of streamline flow of incompressible and non viscous fluid (ideal fluid) through a tube, total energy (sum of pressure energy, potential energy and kinetic energy) per unit volume of fluid is same at all points.

Venturimeter, a device used to measure rate of flow of fluid, works on Bernoulli's theorem.

9. Elasticity

Elasticity : Elasticity is the property of material of a body by virtue of which the body acquires its original shape and size after the removal of deforming force.

Elastic Limit : Elastic limit is the maximum value of deforming force upto which a material shows elastic property and above which the material looses its elastic property.

Stress: The restoring force per unit area set up inside the body subjected to deforming force is called stress.

Strain : The relative change in dimension or shape of a body which is subjected to stress is called strain.

It is measured by ratio of change in length to the original length (logitudional strain), change in volume to original volume (volume strain).

Hooke's law : Under elastic limit, stress is proportional to strain

i.e. stress $\propto$ strain or $\dfrac{\text{stress}}{\text{strain}} = E$ (constant)

E is called elastic constant or modulus of elasticity. Its value is different for different material. Its SI unit is Nm^{-2} also called pascal.

Elastic constant is of three types :

(i) Young's modulus of elasticity $Y = \dfrac{\text{Logitudinal stress}}{\text{Logitudinal strain}}$

(ii) Bulk modulus of elasticity $K = \dfrac{\text{Volume stress}}{\text{Volume strain}}$

(iii) Rigidity modulus $(\eta) = \dfrac{\text{Tangential (or shear) stress}}{\text{Shear strain}}$

10. Simple Harmonic Motion

Periodic Motion : Any motion which repeats itself after regular interval of time is called periodic or harmonic motion. Motion of hands of a clock, motion of earth around the sun, motion of the needle of a sewing machine are the examples of periodic motion.

Oscillatory Motion : If a particles repeats its motion after a regular time interval about a fixed point, motion is said to be oscillatory or vibratory, i.e. oscillatory motion is a constrained periodic motion between precisely fixed limits. Motion of piston in an automobile engine, motion of balance wheel of a watch are the examples of oscillatory motion.

Time Period : Time taken in one complete oscillation is called time period.

Or, Time after which motion is repeated is called time period.

Frequency = Frequency is the no. of oscillations completed by oscillating body in unit time interval. Its SI unit is Hertz.

If n = frequency, T = time period, then $nT = 1$

Simple Harmonic Motion : If a particle repeats its motion about a fixed point after a regular time interval in such a way that at any moment the acceleration of the particle is directly proportional to its displacement from the fixed point at that moment and is always directed towards the fixed point then the motion of the particle is called simple harmonic motion.

The fixed point is called mean point or equilibrium point.

Characteristics of SHM

When a particle executing SHM passes through the mean position :
(i) No force acts on the particle.
(ii) Acceleration of the particle is zero.
(iii) Velocity is maximum.
(iv) Kinetic energy is maximum.
(v) Potential energy is zero.

When a particle executing SHM is at the extreme end, then :
(i) acceleration of the particle is maximum.
(ii) Restoring force acting on particle is maximum.
(iii) Velocity of particle is zero.
(iv) Kinetic energy of particle is zero.
(v) Potential energy is maximum.

Simple Pendulum : If a point mass is suspended from a fixed support with the help of a massless and inextensible string, the arrangement is called simple pendulum. The above is an ideal definition. Practically a simple pendulum is made by suspending a small ball (called bob) from a fixed support with the help of a light string.

If the bob of a simple pendulum is slightly displaced from its mean position and then released, it starts oscillating in simple harmonic motion. Time period of oscillation of a simple pendulum is given as

$$T = 2\pi\sqrt{\frac{l}{g}}$$ where l is the effective length of the pendulum and g is the

acceleration due to gravity.

11. Wave

➪ A wave is a disturbance which propagates energy from one place to the other without the transport of matter.

Waves are broadly of two types
(i) Mechanical Wave   (ii) Non-mechanical wave

➪ **Mechanical Wave :** The waves which require material medium (solid, liquid or gas) for their propagation are called mechanical waves or elastic wave.

Mechanical wave are of two types:

(i) **Longitudinal wave :** If the particles of the medium vibrate in the direction of propagation of wave, the wave is called longitudinal wave.

Waves on springs or sound waves in air are examples of longitudual waves.

(ii) **Transverse wave :** If the particles of the medium vibrate perpendicular to the direction of propagation of wave, the wave is called transverse wave.

Waves on strings under tension, waves on the surface of water are examples of transverse waves.

⇨ **Non-mechanical waves or electromagnetic waves :** The waves which do not require medium for their propagation i.e. which can propagate even through the vacuum are called non mechanical wave.

Light, heat are the examples of non-mechanical wave. In fact all the electromagnetic waves are non-mechanical.

⇨ All the electromagnetic wave consists of photon.

⇨ The wavelength range of electromagnetic wave is 10^{-14} m to 10^4 m.

Properties of electromagnetic waves

(i) They are neutral.

(ii) They propagate as transverse wave.

(iii) They propagate with the velocity of light.

(iv) They contains energy and momentum.

(v) Their concept was introduced by Maxwell.

Following waves are not electromagnetic

(i) Cathode rays (ii) Canal rays (iii) α rays (iv) β rays (v) Sound wave (vi) Ultrasonic wave

Some Important Electromagnetic Waves

Electro-magnetic Waves	Discoverer	Wavelength range (in meter)	Frequency range
y-Rays	Henry Becqueral	10^{-14} to 10^{-10}	10^{20} to 10^{18}
X-Rays	W.Rontgen	10^{-10} to 10^{-8}	10^{18} to 10^{16}
Ultra-violet rays	Ritter	10^{-8} to 10^{-7}	10^{16} to 10^{14}
Visible radiation	Newton	3.9×10^{-7} to 7.8×10^{-7}	10^{14} to 10^{12}
Infra-red rays	Hershel	7.8×10^{-7} to 7.8×10^{-3}	10^{12} to 10^{10}
Short radio waves or Hertz Hertzian Waves	Heinrich	10^{-3} to 1	10^{10} to 10^8
Long Radio Waves	Marcony	1 to 10^4	10^8 to 10^6

Note: Electromagnetic waves of wavelength range 10^{-3} m to 10^{-2} m are called microwaves.

Phase of vibration : Phase of vibration of a vibrating particle at any instant is the physical quantity which express the position as well as direction of motion of the particle at that instant with respect to its equilibrium (mean) position.

Amplitude : Amplitude is defined as the maximum displacement of the vibrating particle on either side from the equilibrium position.

Wavelength : Wavelength is the distance between any two nearest particle of the medium, vibrating in the same phase. It is denoted by the Greek letter *lembda*. (λ).

In transverse wave distance between two consecutive crests or troughs and in longitudinal wave, distance between two consecutive compressions or rarefaction is equal to wavelength.

Relation between wavelength, frequency and velocity of wave

Velocity of wave = frequency × wavelength or, $v = n\lambda$.

12. Sound Wave

⇨ Sound waves are longitudinal mechanical waves.

⇨ According to their frequency range, longitudinal mechanical waves are divided into the following categories :

1. **Audible or Sound Waves** : The longitudinal mechanical waves which lie in the frequency range 20 Hz to 20000 Hz are called audible or sound waves. These waves are sensitive to human ear. These are generated by the vibrating bodies such as tuning fork, vocal cords etc.

2. **Infrasonic Waves** : The longitudinal mechanical waves having frequencies less than 20Hz are called Infrasonic. These waves are produced by sources of bigger size such as earth quakes, volcanic eruptions, ocean waves and by elephants and whales.

3. **Ultrasonic Waves** : The longitudinal mechanical waves having frequencies greater than 20000 Hz are called ultrasonic waves. Human ear can not detect these waves. But certain creatures like dog, cat,. bat, mosquito can detect these waves. Bat not only detect but also produce ultrasonic.

Ultrasonic waves can be produced by Galton's whistle or Hartman's generator or by the high frequency vibrations of a quartz crystal under an alternating electric field (Piezo - electric effect) or by the vibrations of a ferromagnetic rod under an alternating magnetic field (Magnetostriction)

Applications of Ultrasonic Waves

1. For sending signals.
2. For measuring the depth of sea.
3. For cleaning cloths, aeroplanes and machinery parts of clocks.
4. For removing lamp-shoot from the chimney of factories.
5. In sterilizing of a liquid .
6. In Ultrasonography.

Speed of Sound

⇨ Speed of sound is different in different mediums. In a medium, the speed of sound basically depends upon elasticity and density of medium.

⇨ Speed of sound is maximum in solids and minimum in gases.

⇨ When sound enters from one medium to another medium, its speed and wavelength changes but frequency remains unchanged.

⇨ In a medium, the speed of sound is independent of frequency.

Effect of pressure on speed of sound: The speed of sound is independent of pressure i.e. speed remains unchanged by the increase or decrease of pressure.

Effect of Temperature on speed of sound : The speed of sound increases with the increase of temperature of the medium. The speed of sound in air increases by 0.61 m/s when the temperature is increased by 1°C.

Effect of humidity on speed of sound : The speed of sound is more in humid air than in dry air because the density of humid air is less than the density of dry air.

Characteristics of Sound Waves : Sound waves have the following three characteristics.

Speed of sound in different mediums

Medium	Speed of sound (in m/s)
Carbondioxide	260
Air (0°C)	332
Air (20°C)	343
Steam (at l00°C)	405
Helium	965
Alcohal	1213
Hydrogen	1269
Mercury	1450
Water (20°C)	1482
Sea water	1533
Copper	3560
Iron	5130
Glass	5640
Granite	6000
Aluminium	6420

1. **Intensity :** Intensity of sound at any point in space is defined as amount of energy passing normally per unit area held around that point per unit time. SI Unit of Intensity is watt/m^2.

   Intensity of sound at a point is,

   (i) inversely proportional to the square of the distance of point from the source.

   (ii) directly proportional to square of amplitude of vibration, square of frequency and density of the medium .

Due to intensity, a sound appears loud or faint to the ear. Actually, the sensation of a sound perceived in ear is measured by another term called **loudness** which depends on intensity of sound and sensitiveness of the ear. Unit of loudness is **bel**. A practical unit of loudness is decibel (dB) which of equal to 1/l0th of bel. Another unit of loudness is **phon**.

2. **Pitch :** Pitch is that characteristic of sound which distinguishes a sharp or shrill sound from a grave (dull or flat) sound. Pitch depends upon frequency. Higher the frequency, higher will be the pitch and shriller will be the sound. Lower the frequency, lower will be the pitch and grave will be the sound.

3. **Quality** : Quality is that characteristic of sound which enables us to distinguish between sounds produced by two sources having the same intensity and pitch. The quality depends upon number, frequency and relative intensities of overtones.

Echo : The sound waves received after being reflected from a high tower or mountains is called echo.

➪ To hear echo, the minimum distance between the observer and reflector should be 17 m (16.6 m)

➪ Persistence of ear (effect of sound on ear) is 1/10 sec.

➪ Due to refraction, sound is heard at longer distances in nights than in day.

Resonance : If the frequency of imposed periodic force is equal to the natural frequency of a body, the body oscillates with a very large amplitude. This phenomenon is called resonance .

Interference of sound : The modification or redistribution of energy at a point due to superposition of two (or, more) sound waves of same frequency is called interference of sound.

If two waves meet at a point in same phase, intensity of sound is maximum at that point. Such type of interference is called constructive interference. Similarly, if the two waves meet at a point in opposite phase, intensity of sound at that point is minimum. Such type of interference is called destructive interference.

Diffraction of sound : Wavelength of sound is of the order of 1 m. If an obstacle of that range appears in the path of sound, sound deviates at the edge of obstacle and propagates forward. This phenomenon is called diffraction of sound.

Doppler's Effect : If there is a relative motion between source of sound and observer, the apparent frequency of sound heard by the observer is different from the actual frequency of sound emitted by the source. This phenomenon is called Doppler's effect.

When the distance between the source and observer decreases, the apparent frequency increases and vice-versa.

Mach Number : It is defined as the ratio of speed of sound source to the speed of sound in the same medium under the same condition of temperature and pressure.

➪ If Mach number > 1, body is called supersonic.

➪ If Mach number > 5, body is called hypersonic.

➪ If Mach number < 1, the body (source) is said to be moving with subsonic speed.

Shock waves : A body moving with supersonic speed in air leaves behind it a conical region of disturbance which spreads continuously. Such a disturbance is called shock wave. This wave carries huge energy and may even make cracks in window panes or even damage a building.

Bow Waves : When a motor boat in a sea travels faster than sound, then waves just like shock-waves are produced on the surface of water. These waves are called bow waves.

13. Heat

Heat is that form of energy which flows from one body to other body due to difference is temperature between the bodies. The amount of heat . contained in a body depends upon the mass of the body.

⇨ If W work is performed and heat produced is H then $W/H = J$ or, $W = JH$ where J is a constant called Mechanical Equivalent of Heat. Its value is 4.186 joule/Calorie. It means if 4.186 joule of work is performed, 1 calorie of heat is consumed.

Units of Heat

C.G .S unit : calorie = It is the amount of heat required to raise the temperature of 1 g of pure water through 1°C.

International calorie : It is the amount of heat required to raise the temperature of 1g of pure water from 14.5°C to 15.5°C.

F.P.S. unit : B.Th.U (British Thermal Unit) = It is the amount of heat required to raise the temp. of 1 pound of pure water through 1°F.

Relations between different units :

1 B.Th.U = 252 calorie	1 calorie = 4.186 joule
1 Therm = 10^5 B.Th.U	1 pound calorie = 453.6 calorie

Temperature : Temperature is that physical cause which decides the direction of flow of heat from one body to other body. Heat energy always flows from body at higher temperature to body at lower temperature.

Measurement of Temperature

Thermometer : The device which measures the temperature of a body is called thermometer.

Scales of temperature measurement

To measure temperature two fixed points are taken on each thermometer. One of the fixed points is the freezing point of water or ice as lower fixed point (LFP). The other fixed point is the boiling point of water or steam as upper fixed print (UFP).

The temperatures of these fixed points, the no. of fundamental interval between the two fixed points on different temperature scales is shown by the table given below :

	Celsius	Fahrenheit	Reaumur	Kelvin	Rankine
UFP	100°C	212°F	80°F	373.15K	672°Ra
no. of fundamental interval	↑ 100 ↓	↑ 180 ↓	↑ 80 ↓	↑ 100 ↓	↑ 180 ↓
LFP	0°C	32°F	0°R	273.15K	492°Ra
Absolute zero	–273.15°C	–459.6°F	–218.4°R	0K	0°Ra

Relation between Temperature on different scales

$$\frac{C-0}{100} = \frac{F-32}{180} = \frac{R-0}{80} = \frac{K-273}{100} = \frac{Ra-492}{180}$$

⇨ Celsius was initially known as centigrade.
⇨ While expressing temperature on kelvin scale 0° (degree) is not used.
⇨ Freezing point (F.P.) of mercury is –39°C. Hence to measure temperature below this temperature, alcohal thermometer is used. F.P. of alcohal is –115°C.

Range of different thermometers
Mercury Thermometer : from –30°C to 350°C
Constant volume gas thermometer: from –200°C to 500°C (with H), below- 200°C upto –268°C (with He) above 1000 °C upto 1600 °C (with N_2 gas and bulb of glazed porcelain)
Platinum resistance thermometer : from –200°C to 1200°C
Thermocouple thermometer : from –200°C to 1600°C

Total Radiation Pyrometer
When a body is at high temperature, it glows brightly and the radiation emitted by the body is directly proportional to the fourth power of absolute temperature of the body. Radiation pyrometer measures the temperature of a body by measuring the radiation emitted by the body.

This thermometer is not put in contact with the body. But it can not measure temperature below 800°C because at low temperature emission of radiation is very small and can not be detected.

Specific Heat Capacity : Specific heat capacity of a material is the

Specific Heat Capacities of different materials (J/kg K)	
Water	4200
Ice	2100
Iron	460
K. Oil	210
Mercury	140
Lead	130

amount of heat required to raise the temperature of unit mass of substance through 1°. Its SI unit is Joule/kilogram kelvin (J/kg.k)

⇨ One calorie of heat is required to raise the temperature of 1 gram of water through 1°C. Hence specific heat capacity of water is 1 cal/gram°C.

1 calorie/gram°C = 4200 Joule/kg kelvin.

Thermal Expansion

When a body is heated its length, surface area and volume increase. The increase in length, area and volume with the increase in temperature are measured in terms of coefficient of linear expansion or linear expansivity (α), coefficient of superficial expansion or superficial expansivity (β) and coefficient ofcubical expansion or cubical expansivity (γ).

Relation between α, β and γ

$\alpha : \beta : \gamma = 1 : 2 : 3$ or, $\beta = 2\alpha$ and $\gamma = 3\alpha$

Anomalous expansion of water : Almost every liquid expands with the increase in temperature. But when temperature of water is increased from 0°C to 4°C, its volume decreases. If the temperature is increased above 4°C, its volume starts increasing. Clearly, density of water is maximum at 4°C.

Transmission of Head : The transfer of heat from one place to other place is called transmission of heat. There are three modes of heat transfer– (i) conduction, (ii) convection and (iii) radiation.

Conduction : In this process, heat is transferred from one place to other place by the successive vibrations of the particles of the medium without bodily movement of the particles of the medium. In solids, heat transfer takes place by conduction.

Convection : In this process, heat is transferred by the actual movement of particles of the movement from one place to other place. Due to movement of particles, a current of particles set up which is called convection current.

In liquids and gases, heat transfer takes place by convection.

⇨ Earth's atmosphere is heated by convection.

Radiation : In this method transfer of heat takes place with the speed of light without affecting the intervening medium.

Newton's law of cooling : The rate of loss of heat by a body is directly proportional to the difference in temperature between the body and the surrounding.

Kirchhoff's law : According to Kirchhoff's law, the ratio of emissive power to absorptive power is same for all surfaces at the same temperature and is equal to emissive power of black body at that temperature.

Kirchhoff's law signifies that good absorbers are good emitter.

If a shining metal ball with some black spot on its surface is heated to a high temperature and seen in dark, the shining ball becomes dull but the black spots shines brilliantly, because black spot absorbs radiation during heating and emit in dark.

Stefan's law : The radiant energy emitted by a black body per unit area per unit time (i.e. emissive power) is directly proportional to the fourth power of its absolute temperature.

i.e. $E \propto T^4$ or, $E = \sigma T^4$

where σ is a constant called Stefan's constant.

Change of State

Any material can remain in any of its three states (solid, liquid and gas). To change the substance from one state to other state is called change of state. For this either substance is heated or heat is extracted from the substance. Change of state takes place at a fixed temp.

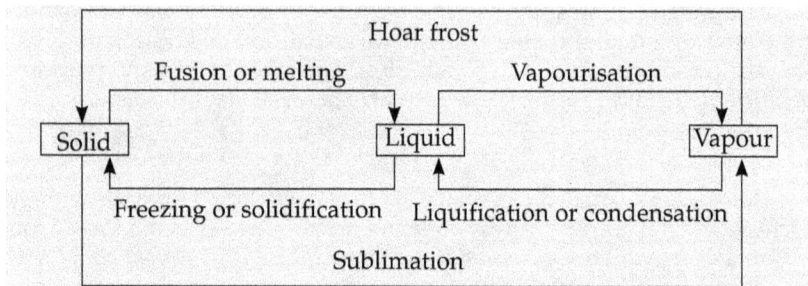

Fusion : The process by which a substance is changed from solid state to liquid state is called fusion. Fusion takes place at a fixed temperature called melting point (M.P.)

Freezing: The process by which a substance is changed from liquid state to solid state is called freezing. Freezing takes at a fixed temperature called freezing point. (F.P.) For a substance M.P.= F.P.

➪   M.P. of a substance changes with the change in pressure. Melting point of substances which contracts in the process of fusion (as ice) decreases with the increase in pressure. Melting point of substances which expands in the process of fusion (as wax) increases with the increase in pressure.

➪   With the addition of impurity (as salt in ice), melting point of a substance decreases.

Vapourisation: The process by which a substance is changed from liquid state to vapour state is called vapourisation.

Vapourisation takes place by two methods: (i) Evaporation & (ii) Boiling or Ebullition

Evaporation : The process of vapourisation which takes place only from the exposed surface of liquid and that at all temperatures is called evaporation.

Evaporation causes cooling. This is why water in a earthed pot gets cooled in summer.

Boiling : The process of vapourisation which takes place at a fixed temperature and from whole part of liquid is called boiling.

The temperature at which boiling takes place is called boiling point .

Condensation : The process by which a substance is changed from vapour state to liquid state is called condensation.

➪   Boiling point of a liquid increases with the increase in pressure.

➪   Boiling point of a liquid increases with the addition of impurity.

Latent heat or heat of transformation

The amount of heat required to change the state of unit mass of substance at constant temperature is called latent heat.

If Q heat is required to change the state of a substance of mass m at constant temperature and L is the latent heat, then $Q = mL$.

S.I unit of latent heat is Joule/kilogram. Any material has two types of latent heat.

(i) **Latent heat of fusion :** It is the amount of heat energy required to convert unit mass a substance from solid state to liquid state at its melting point. It is also the amount of heat released by unit mass of liquid when changed into solid at its freezing point.

(ii) **Latent heat of vapourisation :** It is the amount of heat required to change unit mass of a substance from liquid state to vapour state at its boiling point. It is also the amount of heat released when unit mass of a vapour is changed into liquid.

Latent heat of water

Latent Heat	in Cal/g	J/kg
of fusion	80	336×10^3
of vapourisation	540	2256×10^3

Sublimation: Sublimation is the process of conversion of a solid directly into vapour.

⇨ Sublimation takes place when boiling point is less than melting point.

⇨ Sublimation is shown by camphor or ice in vacuum.

Hoar Frost : Hoar frost is just the reverse process of sublimation i.e. it is the process of direct conversion of vapour into solid.

⇨ Steam produces more severe burn than water at same temperature because internal energy of steam is more than that of water at same temperature.

Relative Humidity : Relative humidity is defined as the ratio of amount of water vapour present in a given volume of atmosphere to the amount of water vapour required to saturate the same volume at same temperature.

The ratio is multiplied by 100 to express the relative humidity in percentage.

⇨ Relative humidity is measured by Hygrometer.

⇨ Relative humidity increases with the increase of temperature.

Air conditioning : For healthy and favourable atmosphere of human being, the conditions are as follows

(i) **Temperature :** from 23°C to 25°C.

(ii) **Relative humidity :** from 60% to 65%.

(iii) **Speed of air :** from 0.75 meter/minute to 2.5 meter/minute.

Thermodynamics

First law of thermodynamics : Heat energy given to a system is used in the following two ways :

(i) In increasing the temperature and hence internal energy of the system.

(ii) In doing work by the system.

If ΔQ = heat energy given to the system

ΔU = Increase in the internal energy of the system.

ΔW = work done by the system

Then, $\Delta Q = \Delta U + \Delta W$ is the mathematical statement of first law of thermodynamics.

➪ First law of thermodynamics is equivalent to principle of conservation of energy.

Isothermal Process : If the changes are taking place in a system in such a way that temperature of the system remains constant throughout the change, then the process is said to be an isothermal.

Adiabatic Process : If the changes are taking place in a system in such a way that there is no exchange of heat energy between the system and the surrounding, then the process is said to be an adiabatic process.

➪ If carbon dioxide is suddenly expanded, it is changed into dry ice. This is an example of adiabatic process.

Second Law of Thermodynamics : The first law of thermodynamics guarantees that in a thermodynamic process, energy will be conserved. But this law does not tell whether a given process in which energy is conserved will take place or not. The second law of thermodynamics gives the answer.

Through this law can be stated in many forms, the following two forms are worth mentioning :

Kelvin's statement : Whole of the heat can never be converted into work.

Clausius statement : Heat by itself can not flow from a colder body to a hotter body.

Heat Engine : Heat energy is a device which converts heat energy into mechanical work continuously through a cyclic process. Every heat engine basically consists of the three parts: (i) source (a hot body) (ii) sink (a cold body) and (iii) a working substance.

Heat engine may be devided into two types :

(i) **Internal Combustion Engine :** In this engine, heat is produced in the engine itself. *Example* :Otto engine or petrol engine (efficiency = 52%), Diesel engine (efficiency = 64%)

(ii) **External Cumbustion Engine :** In this engine heat is produced outside the engine. Steam engine is an example of external cumbustion engine. (efficiency = 20%)

Refrigerator or Heat Pump : A refrigerator is an apparatus which transfers heat energy from cold to a hot body at the expanse of energy supplied by an external agent. The working substance here is called refrigerant.

In actual refrigerator, vapours of freon (CCl_2F_2) acts as refrigerant.

14. Light

Light is a form of energy which is propagated as electromagnetic waves. In the spectrum of electromagnetic waves it lies between ultra-violet and infra-red region and has wavelength between 3900 A° to 7800 A°.

⇨ Electromagnetic waves are transverse, hence light is transverse wave.

⇨ Wave nature of light explains rectilinear propagation, reflection, refraction, interference, diffraction and polarisation of light.

⇨ The phenomena like photo electric effect, compton effect are not explained on the basis of wave nature of light. These phenomena are explained on the basis of quantum theory of light as proposed by Einstein.

⇨ In quantum theory, light is regarded as a packet or bundle of energy called photon. Photon is associated with it an energy E where $E = hv$.

⇨ Clearly light behaves as wave and particle both. Thus light has dual nature.

⇨ Speed of light was first measured by Roemer. (1678 AD).

⇨ Speed of light is maximum in vacuum and air (3×10^8 m/s)

Refractive index : R.I. of a medium is defined as the ratio of speed of light in vacuume to the speed of light in the medium.

$$\mu = \frac{c}{v} = \frac{\text{Speed of light in vacuum}}{\text{Speed of light in the medium}}$$

⇨ Speed of light is different in different media. Velocity of light is large in a medium which has small refractive index.

Speed of light in different mediums

Medium	Speed of light (m/s)	Medium	Speed of light (m/s)
Vacuum	3×10^8	Glass	2×10^8
Water	2.25×10^8	Terpentine oil	2.04×10^8
Rock salt	1.96×10^8	Nylon	1.96×10^8

⇨ Light takes 8 minute 19 second (499 second) to reach from sun to earth.

⇨ The light reflected from moon takes 1.28 second to reach earth.

Luminous bodies : Those object which emit light by themselves are called luminous bodies.

e.g.–sun, stars, electric bulb etc.

Non-luminous bodies: Those objects which do not emit light by themselves but are visible by the light falling on them emitted by self luminous bodies are called non-luminous bodies.

A material can be classified as :

(i) **Transparent:** The substances which allow most of the incident light to pass through them are called transparent, e.g. glass, water.

(ii) Translucent: The substances which allow a part of incident light to pass through them are called translucent bodies e.g. oiled paper.

(iii) Opaque : The substances which do not allow the incident light to pass through them are called opaque bodies, e.g., mirror, metal, wood etc.

Reflection of light : Light moving in one medium when falls at the Surface of another medium, part of light returns back to the same medium. This phenomenon of returning back of light in the first medium at the interface of two media is known as reflection of light.

Laws of reflection

(i) The incident ray, reflected ray and normal to the reflecting surface at the incident point all lie in the same plane,

(ii) The angle of reflection is equal to the angle of incidence.

Reflection from plane mirror

(i) The image is virtual, laterally inverted.

(ii) The size of image is equal to that of object.

(iii) The distance of image from the mirror is equal to distance of object from the mirror.

(iv) If an object moves towards (or away from) a plane mirror with speed v, relative to the object the image moves towards (or away) with a speed $2v$.

(v) If a plane mirror is rotated by an angle θ, keeping the incident ray fixed, the reflected ray is rotated by an angle 2θ.

(vi) To see his full image in a plane mirror, a person requires a mirror of at least half of his height.

(vii) If two plane mirrors are inclined to each other at an angle θ the number of images (n) of a point object formed are determined as follows:

(a) If $\dfrac{360}{\theta}$ is even integer, then $n = \dfrac{360}{\theta} - 1$

(b) If $\dfrac{360}{\theta}$ is odd integer,

then $n = \dfrac{360}{\theta} - 1$ *for the object is symmetrically placed, and*

$n = \dfrac{360}{\theta}$ *for the object is not symmetrically placed.*

(c) If $\dfrac{360}{\theta}$ is a fraction then n is equal to integral part.

Reflection from spherical mirror

Spherical mirror are of two types (i) Concave mirror and (ii) Convex mirror

Position & nature of image formed by a spherical mirror

Position of object	Position of image	Size of image in comparison to Object	Nature of image
Concave mirror			
At infinity	At Focus	Highly diminished	Real, inverted
Between infinity and centre of curvature	Between focus and centre of curvature	Diminished	Real, inverted
At centre curvature	At centre of curvature	Of same size	Real, inverted
Between focus and centre of curvature	Between centre of curvature and infinity	Enlarged	Real, inverted
At focus	At infinity	Highly enlarged	Real, inverted
Between focus and pole	Behind the mirror	Enlarged	Virtual, erect
Convex mirror			
At infinity	At Focus	Highly diminished	Virtual, erect
In front of mirror	Between pole and focus	Diminished	Virtual, erect

Note : *Image formed by a convex mirror is always virtual, erect and diminished.*

Uses of Concave mirror :
(i)   As a shaving glass.
(ii) As a reflector for the head lights of a vehicle, search light.
(iii) In opthalmoscope to examine eye, ear, nose by doctors.
(iv) In solar cookers.

Uses of Convex mirror :
(i)   As a rear view mirror in vehicle because it provides the maximum rear field of view and image formed is always erect.
(ii) In sodium reflector lamp.

Refraction of light: When a ray of light propagating in a medium enters the other medium, it deviates from its path. This phenomenon of change in the direction of propagation of light at the boundary when it passes from one medium to other medium is called refraction of light.

When a ray of light enters from rarer medium to denser medium (as from water to glass) it deviates towards the normal drawn on the boundary of two media at the incident point. Similarly in passing from denser to rarer medium, a ray deviates away from the normal. If light is incident normally on the boundary i.e. parallel to normal, it enters the second medium undeviated.

Laws of refraction

   (i)   Incident ray, refracted ray and normal drawn at incident point always lie in the same plane.

  (ii) Snell's law : For a given colour of light, the ratio of sine of angle of incidence to the sine of angle of refraction is a constant,

$$\text{i.e. } \frac{\sin i}{\sin r} = {}^1\mu_2 \text{ (constant)}$$

This constant ${}^1\mu_2$ is called refractive index of second medium with respect to the first medium.

➭   Absolute refractive index of a medium is defined as the ratio of speed of light in free space (vacuum) to that in the given medium.

$$\text{i.e. absolute refractive index } (\mu) = \frac{\text{Speed of light in vacuum}}{\text{Speed of light in the medium}}$$

➭   The refractive index of a medium is different for different colours. The refractive index of a medium decreases with the increase in wavelength of light. Hence refractive index of a medium is maximum for violet colour of light and minimum for red colour of light.

➭   The refractive index of a medium decreases with the increase in temperature. But this variation is very small.

➭   When a ray of light enters from one medium to other medium, its frequency and phase donot change but wavelength and velocity change.

Some illustrations of Refraction

   (i)   Bending of a linear object when it is partially dipped in a liquid to the surface of the liquid.

  (ii) Twinkling of stars.

 (iii) Oval shape of sun in the morning and evening.

 (iv) An object in a denser medium when seen from a rarer medium appears to be at a smaller distance.

   This is way (a) A fish in a pond when viewed from air appears to be at a smaller depth them actual depth (b) A coin at the base of a vessel filled water appears raised.

   Critical angle : In case of propagation of light from denser to rarer medium through a plane boundary, critical angle is the angle of incidence for which angle of refraction is 90°.

   Total Internal Reflection : If light is propagating from denser medium towards the rarer medium and angle of incidence is more than critical angle, then the light incident on the boundary is reflected back in the denser medium, obeying the laws of reflection. This phenomenon is called total internal reflection as total light energy is reflected, no part is absorbed or transmitted.

➪ For total internal reflection,
  (i) Light must be propagating from denser to rarer medium.
  (ii) Angle of incidence must exceeds the critical angle.

Illustration's of total internal reflection
  (i) Sparkling of diamond
  (ii) Mirage and looming.
  (iii) Shining of air bubble in water.
  (iv) Increase in duration of sun's visibility – The sun becomes visible even before sun rise and remains visible even after sunset due to total internal reflection of light.
  (v) Shining of a smoked ball or a metal ball on which lamp soot is deposited when dipped in water.
  (vi) **Optical Fibre:** Optical fibre consists of thousands of strands of a very fine quality glass or quartz (of refractive index 1.7), each strand coated with a layer of material of lower refractive index (1.5). In it, light is propagated along the axis of fibre through multiple total internal reflection, even though the fibre is curved, without loss of energy.

Applications :
  (i) For transmitting optical signals and the two dimensional pictures.
  (ii) For transmitting electrical signals by first converting them to light.
  (iii) For visualising the internal sites of the body by doctors in endoscopy.

Refraction of Light Through Lens
➪ Lens is a section of transparent refractive material of two surfaces of definite geometrical shape of which one surface must be spherical. Lens is generally of two types : (i) Convex lens (ii) Concave lens.
➪ When a lens is thicker at the middle than at the edges, it is called a convex lens or a converging lens. When the lens is thicker at the edges than in the middle, it is called as concave lens or diverging lens.
➪ Some terms regarding a lens.

Convex Lens
C_2 F_1 O F_2 C_1

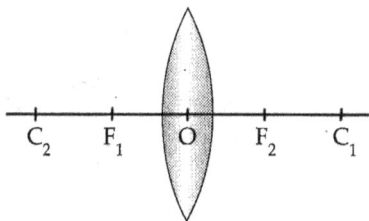

O – Optical Centre
C_1C_2 –Principal axis

Concave lens
C_1 F_2 O F_1 C_2

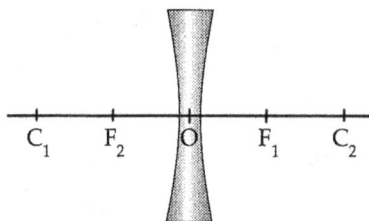

F_1 – First Focus
F_2 – Second Focus

Power of a lens

⇨ Power of a lens is its capacity to deviate a ray. It is measured as the reciprocal of the focal length in meters, i.e. $P = \dfrac{1}{f}$

SI Unit of power is dioptre (D).

⇨ Power of a convex lens is positive and that of a concave lens is negative.

⇨ If two lenses are placed in contact, then the power of combination is equal to the sum of powers of individual lenses.

Change in the power of a lens : If a lens is dipped in a liquid, its focal length and power both change. This change depends upon the refractive indices of lens and the liquid. If a lens of refractive index μ is dipped in a liquid of refractive index μ', then the following three situations are possible.

(i) $\mu > \mu'$ i.e. lens is dipped in a liquid of smaller refractive index like a lens of glass ($\mu = 1.5$) is dipped in water (($\mu' = 1.33$), then the focal length of the lens increases and the power of the lens decreases.

(ii) $\mu = \mu'$ i.e. lens is dipped in a liquid of equal refractive index then the focal length of the lens becomes infinite i.e. its power becomes zero. The lens and the liquid behave as a single medium.

(iii) $\mu < \mu'$ i.e. lens is dipped in a liquid of higher refractive index the focal length increases i.e. power decreases as well as the nature of the lens also changes i.e. convex lens behaves as concave lens and vice-versa. For example, an air bubble trapped in water or glass appears as convex but behaves as concave lens. Similarly a convex lens of glass ($\mu = 1.5$) when dipped in carbon disulphide ($\mu' = 1.68$), it behaves as a concave lens.

Formation of images by lenses

Position of object	Position of image	Size of image	Nature of image
Convex Lens			
At infinity	At Focus	Highly, diminished	Real, inverted
Beyond 2F	Between F and 2F	Diminished	Real, inverted
At 2F	At 2F	Of same size	Real, inverted
Between F and 2F	Beyond 2F	Enlarged	Real, inverted
At F	At infinity	Highly enlarged	Real, inverted
Between optical centre and F	The same side as in the object	Enlarged	Virtual and erect

Concave Lens

At infinity	At focus	Highly diminished	Virtual and erect
Between lens and infinity	Between lens and F on the same side	Diminished	Virtual and erect

Dispersion of Light: When a ray of white light (or a composite light) is passed through a prism, it gets splitted into its constituent colours. This phenomenon is called dispersion of light. The coloured pattern obtained on a screen after dispersion of light is called spectrum.

↻ The dispersion of light is due to different deviation suffered by different colours of light. The deviation is maximum for violet colour and minimum for red colour of light. The different colours appeared in the spectrum are on the following order, violet, indigo, blue, green, yellow, orange and red. (VIBGYOR)

↻ The dispersion of light is due to different velocities of light of different colours in a medium. As a result, the refractive index of a medium is different for different colours of light.

↻ The velocity of light in a medium is maximum for that colour for which refractive index is minimum. Clearly, the velocity of violet colour of light is minimum in a medium and retroactive index of that medium is maximum for violet colour. Similarly, the velocity of light in a medium is maximum for red colour and refractive index of that medium is minimum for red colour.

Rainbow : Rainbow is the coloured display in the form of an arc of a circle hanging in the sky observed during or after a little drizzle appearing on the opposite side of sun. Rainbow is formed due to dispersion of sun light by the suspended water droplets.

Rainbow is of two types : (i) Primary rainbow (ii) Secondary rainbow

↻ Primary rainbow is formed due to two refractions and one total internal reflection of light falling on the raindrops. In the primary rainbow, the red colour is on the convex side and violet on the concave side. Primary rainbow has an angular width of 2° at an average angle of elevation of 41°.

↻ Secondary rainbow is formed due to two refractions and two internal reflections of light falling on rain drops. The order of colour on the secondary rainbow is in the reverse order and has an angular width of 3.5° at an average elevation of 52.75°. Secondary rainbow is less intense than primary rainbow.

Theory of Colours: Colour is the sensation perceived by the rods in the eye due to light.

Primary Colours : The spectral colours blue, green and red are called primary colours because all the colours can be produced by mixing these in proper proportion.

Blue + Red + Green = White

Secondary Colours : The colour produced by mixing any two primary colours is called a secondary colour. There are three secondary colours yellow, magenta and cyan as

Green + Red = Yellow, Red + Blue = Magenta, Blue + Green = Cyan

When the three secondary colours are mixed, white colour is produced

Yellow + Magenta + Cyan = White

Complementary Colours : Any two colours when added produce white light, are said to be complementary colours. Clearly a secondary colour and the remaining primary colour are complementary colours. Red and cyan, blue and yellow and green and magenta are complementary of each other.

⇨ The different colours and their mixtures are shown by the colour triangle.

⇨ In coloured television, the three primary colours are used.

⇨ **Colour of bodies :** The colour of a body is the colour of light which it reflects or transmits. An object is white, if it reflects all the components of white light and it is black if it absorbs all the light incident over it. This is why a red rose appears red when viewed in white or red light but appears black when viewed in blue or green light.

⇨ How a body will appear in light of different colour can be understood by the following table:

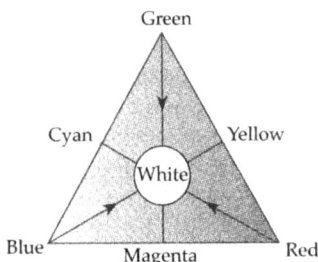

Name of object	In white light	In red light	In green light	In yellow light	In blue light
White paper	White	Red	Green	Yellow	Blue
Red paper	Red	Red	Black	Black	Black
Green paper	Green	Black	Green	Black	Black
Yellow paper	Yellow	Black	Black	Yellow	Black
Blue paper	Blue	Black	Black	Black	Blue

Scattering of light: When light waves fall on small bodies such as dust particles, water particles in suspension, suspended particles in colloidal solution, they are thrown out in all directions. This phenomenon is called scattering of light.

Scattering of light is maximum in case of violet colour and minimum in case of red colour of light.

⇨ Blue colour of sky is due to scattering of light.

⇨ The brilliant red colour of rising and setting sun is due to scattering of light.

Interference of light : When two light waves of exactly the same frequency and a constant phase difference travel in same direction and superimpose then the resultant intensity in the region of superposition is different from the sum of intensity of individual waves. This modification in the intensity of light in the region of superposition is called interference of light. Interference is of two types:

(i) Constructive interference (ii) Destructive interference

Constructive interference : At some points, where the two waves meet is same phase, resultant intensity is maximum. Such interference is called constructive interference.

Destructive interference: At some points, where the two waves meet in opposite phase, resultant intensity is minimum. Such interference is called destructive interference.

Diffraction of light : When light waves fall on a small sized obstacle or a small aperture whose dimension is comparable to the wavelength of light, then there is a departure from the rectilinear propagation and light energy flavours out into the region of geometrical shadow. The spreading of light energy beyond the limit prescribed by rectilinear propagation of light is called diffraction of light. In other words, diffraction is the process by which a beam of light or other systems of wave is spread out as a result of passing through a narrow opening or across an edge.

Polarisation of light : Polarisation is the only phenomenon which proves that light is a transverse wave. Light is an electromagnetic wave in which electric and magnetic field vectors vibrate perpendicular to each other and also perpendicular to the direction of propagation. In ordinary light, the vibrations of elecltric field vector are in every plane perpendicular to the direction of propagation of wave. Polarisation is the phenomenon of restricting the vibrations of a light in a particular direction in a plane perpendicular to the direction of propagation of wave.

⇨ The visible effect of light is only due to electric field vector.

Human Eye

⇨ Least distance of distinct vision is 25 cm.

Defects of human eye and the remedies :

1. **Myopia or short sightedness :** A person suffering from myopia can see the near objects clearly while far objects are not clear.

    Causes : (i) Elongation of eye ball along the axis.

    (ii) Shortening of focal length of eye lens.

    (iii) Over stretching of ciliary muscles beyond the elastic limit.

    Remedy : Diverging lens is used.

2. **Hyperopia or hypermetropia or long sightedness :** A person suffering from hypermetropia can see the distant objects clearly but not the near objects.

    Causes : (i) Shortening of eye ball along the axis.

    (ii) Increase in the focal length of eye lens.

    (iii) Stiffening of ciliary muscles.

    Remedy : A converging lens is sued.

3. **Presbyopia :** This defect is generally found in elderly person. Due to stiffening of ciliary muscles, eye looses much of its accommodating power. As a result distant as well as nearby objects can not be seen. For its remedy two separate lens or a bifocal lens is used.

4. **Astigmatism :** This defect arises due to difference in the radius of curvature of cornea in the different planes. As a result rays from an object in one plane are brought to focus by eye in another plane. For its remedy cylindrical lens is used.

⇨ There are two kinds of vision cells in the retina. They are called rods and cones on account of their peculiar shape. Rods decides the intensity of light where as cones distinguish colour of light.

Simple microscope : This is simply a convex lens of small focal length. The object to be enlarged is placed within the focus of lens.

Magnifying power of a simple microscope is given as

$$M = 1 + \frac{D}{f}$$ where D = 25 cm, f = focal length of lens.

Compound microscope : It consists of two convex lenses coaxially fitted in a hollow tube. The lens facing the object is called objective and the lens towards the eye is called eye piece.

⇨ The aperture of objective is smaller than that of eye piece.

⇨ Both the lenses are of smaller focal lengths. This increases the magnifying power of instrument.

Telescope

Telescopes are used to view distant objects which are not visible to naked eye. Telescope can be divided as astronomical telescope, terrestrial telescope and Galilean telescope.

⇨ Astronomical telescope consists of two convex lenses placed coaxially in a hollow tube. The lens facing the object is called objective and the lens towards the eye is called eye piece.

⇨ The objective has large aperture so that the rays from the object can be easily collected.

⇨ The focal length of objective is larger than that of eye piece.

15. Static Electricity

When two bodies are rubbed together, they acquire the property of attracting light objects like small bits of paper, dust particles etc. The bodies which acquire this property are said to be electrified or charged with electricity.

Charge : Charge is the basic property associated with matter due to which it produces and experiences eletrical and magnetic effects.

⇨ *Benjamin Frankline* named the two types of charges as positive and negative.

⇨ Similar charges repel each other and opposite charges attract each other.

⇨ Charging of bodies takes place due to transfer of electrons from one body to other body.

⇨ A list of materials has been given below. The list is such that any of the material in the list will be positively charged when rubbed with any other material coming later in the list. The other material will naturally be negtively charged.

1.	Fur	2.	Flannel	3.	Shellac	4.	Sealing Wax
5.	Glass	6.	Paper	7.	Silk	8.	Human body
9.	Wood	10.	Metals	11.	India Rubber	12.	Resin
13.	Amber	14.	Sulphur	15.	Ebonite	16.	Gutta Percha

Surface density of charge : Surface density of charge is defined as the amount of charge per unit area on the surface of conductor.
➪ The surface density of charge at a point on the surface of conductor depends upon the shape of conductor and presence of other conductors or insulators near the given conductor.
➪ The surface density of charge at any part of the conductor is inversely proportional to the radius of curvature of the surface of that part.
This is why surface density of charge in maximum at the pointed parts of the condcutor.

Conductor : Conductors are those materials which allow electricity (charge) to pass through themselves.
Examples: (a) Metals like silver, iron, copper (b) Earth (especially the moist part) acts like a huge conductor.
➪ Silver is the best conductor.

Insulator or Dielectric: Insulators are those materials which do not allow electricity to flow through themselves.
Examples : Wood, paper, mica, glass, ebonite.

Coulomb's law : According to Coulomb's law, the force of attraction or repulsion between two point charges at rest is directly proportional to the product of the magnitudes of the charges and inversely proportional to the square of the distance between them. This force acts on the line joining the two charges.

Electric Field : Region in space around a charge or charged body where the charge has its electrical effect is called electric field of the charge.

Electric Field Intensity : Electric field intensity at a point in an electric field is the force experienced by a unit positive charge placed at that point.

Electric Field of hollow conductor
Electric field intensity inside a charged hollow conductor is zero. Charge given to such a conductor (or conductor of any shape) remains on its surface only.
This explains why a hollow conductor acts as an electrostatic shield. It is for this reason that it is safer to sit in a car or bus during lightning.

Electric Potential : Electric potential at a point in an electric field is the work done in bringing a unit positive charge from infinity to that point.
SI unit of electric potential is volt. It is a scalar quantity.

Potential Difference : Work done in bringing a unit positive charge from one point to other point is the potential difference between the two points. Its SI unit is volt and is a scalar quantity.

Electric Capacity : Electric capacity of a conductor is defined as the charge required to increase the potential of the condcutor by unity. If potential of a conductor is increased by V when a charge Q is given to it, capacity of the conductor is Q/V. Its SI unit is farad. (F).

Electrochemical Cell : Electrochemical cell is a device which converts chemical energy into electrical energy.

Cells are basically of two types : (i) Primary cell (ii) Secondary cell.

Primary Cell : In primary cell electrical energy is obtained from the irreversible chemical reaction taking inside the cell. After complete discharge, primary cell becomes unserviceable.

Examples : Voltaic Cell, Leclanche Cell, Daniel Cell, Dry Cell etc.

Secondary Cell : A secondary cell is that which has to be charged at first from an external electric source and then can be used to draw current. Such cells are rechargeable.

➪ Production of electricity by chemical reaction was first discovered by *Allexandro de volta* (voltaic cell is named after him) in 1794. In voltaic cell zinc rod is used as cathode and copper rod is used as anode. These rods are placed in sulphuric acid kept in a glass vessel.

➪ In a *Leclanche cell*, carbon rod acts as anode and zinc rod acts as cathode.

➪ These rods are placed in amonium chloride kept in a glass vessel.

➪ The emf of Leclanche cell is 1.5 volt.

➪ Leclanche cell is used for intermittent works. i.e. works in which continuous electrical energy is not required like electric bell.

➪ In a dry cell, mixture of MnO_2, NH_4Cl and carbon is kept in a zinc vessel. A carbon rod is placed in the mixture which acts as anode. The zinc vessel itself acts as cathode. The emf of dry cell is 1.5 volt.

16. Current Electricity

Electric Current: Electric current is defined as the rate of flow of charge or charge flowing per unit time interval. Its direction is the direction of flow of positive charge. Its SI unit is ampere (A). It is a scalar quantity.

➪ A current of one ampere flowing through a conductor means 6.25×10^{18} electrons are entering at one end or leaving the other end of the conductor in one second.

Resistance : The opposition offered by a conductor to the flow of current through it is called resistance. It arises due to collisions of drifting electrons with the core ions. Its SI unit is ohm.

Ohm's law : If physical conditions like temperature, intensity of light etc. remains unchanged then electric current flowing through a conductor is directly proportional to the potential difference across its ends. If V is the potential difference across the ends of a conductor and I is the current through it, then according to ohm's law $V \propto I$ or, $V = RI$

where R is a constant called resistance of conductor.

Ohmic Resistance: The resistances of such condcutors which obey ohm's law are called ohmic resistance. For example resistance of *manganin* wire.

Non ohmic resistance : The resistances of such materials which do not obey ohm's law are called *non ohmic* resistance.

Example : Resistance of diode valve, resistance of triode valve.

Conductance : Reciprocal of resistance of a conductor is called its conductance i.e.

$$\text{conductance} = \frac{1}{\text{Resistance}}$$

➪ It is denoted by G, and $\left(G = \dfrac{1}{R}\right)$

Its SI unit is ohm^{-1} (also called mho or siemen.)

➪ The resistance of a conductor is directly proportional to its length and inversely proportional to its cross sectional area. i.e. if l and A are respectively length and cross sectional area of a conductor and R is its resistance then $R \propto \dfrac{l}{A}$ or, $R = \rho \dfrac{l}{A}$

where p is a constant of material of conductor called specific resistance or resistivity. Its SI unit is ohm meter.

Specific conductance or conductivity : The reciprocal of resistivity of a conductor is called its conductivity (s). Its SI unit is mho m^{-1} or siemen/meter (sm^{-1})

Combination of Resistance : Various resistances can be combined to form a network mainly in two ways : (i) Series combination (ii) Parallel combination.

➪ In series combination, the equivalent resistance is equal to the sum of the resistances of individual conductors. $(R = R_1 + R_2 + \dots\dots\dots R_n)$

➪ In parallel combination, the reciprocal of equivalent resistance is equal to the sum of the reciprocal of individual resistances.

$$\left(\frac{1}{2} = \frac{1}{R_1} + \frac{1}{R_2} + \dots + \frac{1}{R_n}\right)$$

Electric Power : The rate at which electrical energy is consumed in a circuit is called electric power. Its SI unit is watt.

Kilowatt hour: It is the unit of energy and is equal to the energy consumed in the circuit at the rate of 1 kilowatt (1000 J/s) for 1 hour.

1 kilowatt hour = 3.6 x 10^6 joule

1 kWh is also called board of trade unit.

Ammeter: Ammeter is a device which is used to measure electric current in a circuit. It is connected in series in the circuit.

➪ The resistance of an ideal ammeter is zero.

Voltmeter: Voltmeter is a device used to measure the potential difference between two points in a circuit. It is connected in parallel to the circuit.

⇨ The resistance of an ideal voltmeter is infinite.

Electric fuse : Electric fuse is a protective device used in series with an electric appliance to save it from being damaged due to high current. In general, it is a small conducting wire of alloy of copper, tin and lead having low melting point.

⇨ Pure fuse is made up of tin.

Galvanometer : Galvanometer is a device used to detect and measure electric current in a circuit. It can measure current up to 10^{-6} A.

Shunt : Shunt is a wire of very small resistance. In simple words, galvanometer is an instrument for detecting and measuring small electric currents.

⇨ A galvanometer can be converted into an ammeter by connecting a shunt parallel to it.

⇨ A galvanometer can be converted into a voltmeter by connecting a very high resistance in its series.

Transformer : Transformer is a device which converts low voltage A.C. into high voltage A.C. and high voltage A.C. into low voltage A.C. It is based on electromagnetic induction and can be used only in case of alternating current.

A.C. Dynamo (or generator) : It is device used to convert mechanical energy into electrical energy. It works on the principle of electro-magnetic induction.

Electric motor : It is a device which converts electrical energy into mechanical energy.

Microphone : It converts sound energy into electrical energy and works on the principle of electromagnetic induction. In other words, microscope is an instrument for changing sound waves into electrical energy which may then be amplified, transmitted or recorded.

⇨ The current generated in the power stations are alternating current having voltage 22000 volt or more. In grid substations, with the help of transformer, their voltage is increased up to 132000 volt to minimise loss of energy in long distance transmission.

17. Magnetism

⇨ Magnetism is the property displayed by magnets and produced by the movement of electric charges, which results in objects being attracted or pushed away.

⇨ Magnet is a piece of iron or other materials that can attract iron containing objects and that points north and south when suspended.

⇨ A magnet is characterised by following two properties :

   (i) **Attractive property :** A magnet attracts magnetic substances like iron, cobalt, nickel and some of their alloys like magnetite (Fe_3O_4)

(ii) Directive property : When a magnet is freely suspended, it aligns itself in the geographical north south direction.

⇨ A magnet may be (i) Natural (ii) Artificial

⇨ Natural magnet is oxide of iron. But due to irregular shape, weak magnetism and high brittleness, natural magnets find no use in the laboratory.

⇨ The magnets made by artificial methods are called artificial magnets or man made magnets. They may be of different types like bar magnet, horse shoe magnet, Robinson's ball ended magnet, magnetic needle, electromagnet etc.

⇨ The two points near the two ends of a magnet where the attracting capacity is maximum are called magnetic poles. When a magnet is freely suspended, its one pole always directs towards the north. This pole is called north pole. The other pole is called south pole.

⇨ The imaginary line joining the two poles of a magnet is called magnetic axis of the magnet.

⇨ Similar poles repel each other and dissimilar poles attract each other.

⇨ When a magnetic substance is placed rear a magnet, it gets magnetised due to induction.

Magnetic Field : Region in space around a magnet where the magnet has its magnetic effect is called magnetic field of the magnet.

Intensity of magnetic field or magnetic flux density : Magnetic flux density of a point in a magnetic field is the force experienced by a north pole of unit strength placed at that point. Its SI unit is newton/ampere-meter or weber/meter^2 or tesla (T).

Magnetic lines of force: The magnetic lines of force are imaginary curves which represent a magnetic field graphically. The tangent drawn at any point on the magnetic liens of force gives the direction of magnetic field at that point.

Properties of magnetic liens of force :

(i) Magnetic lines of force are closed curves. Outside the magnet they are from north to south pole and inside the magnet they are from south to north pole.

(ii) Two lines of force near intersect each other.

(iii) If the lines of force are crowded, the field is strong.

(iv) If the liens of force are parallel and equidistant, the field is uniform.

Magnetic Substance : On the basis of magnetic behaviour, substances can be divided into three categories.

(i) Diamagnetic substance: Diamagnetic substances are such substances which when placed in a magnetic field, acquire feeble magnetism opposite to the direction of magnetic field.

Examples : Bismuth, Zinc, Copper, Silver, Gold, Diamond, Water, Mercury, Water etc.

(ii) **Paramagnetic Substance:** Paramagnetic substances are such substances which when placed in a magnetic field acquire a feeble magnetism in the direction of the field.

Examples : Aluminum, Platinum, Manganese, Sodium, Oxygen etc.

(iii) **Ferromagnetic substance :** Ferromagnetic substances are those substance, which when placed in a magnetic field, are strongly magnetised in the direction of field. Examples : Iron, Cobalt, Nickel etc.

Domain : Atoms of ferromagnetic substance have a permanent dipole moment i.e. they behave like a very small magnet. The atoms form a large no. of effective regions called domain in which 10^{18} to 10^{21} atoms have their dipole moment aligned in the same direction. The magnetism in ferromagnetic substance, when placed in a magnetic field, is developed due to these domain by (i) the displacements of boundaries of the domains (ii) the rotation of the domains.

Curie Temperature : As temperature increases, the magnetic property of ferromagnetic substance decreases and above a certain temperature the substance changes into paramagnetic substance. This temperature is called Curie temperature.

⇨ Permanent magnets are made of steel, cobalt steel, ticonal, alcomax and alnico.

⇨ Electromagnets cores of transformers, telephone diaphragms, armatures of dynamos and motors are made of soft iron, mu-metal and stalloy.

Terrestrial Magnetism: Our earth behaves as a powerful magnet whose south pole is near the geographical north pole and whose north pole is near the geographical south pole. The magnetic field of earth of a place is described in the terms of following three elements.

(i) **Declination :** The acute angle between magnetic meridian and geographical meridian at a place is called the angle of declination at that place.

(ii) **Dip or Inclination :** Dip is the angle which the resultant earth's magnetic field at a place makes with the horizontal. At poles and equator, dip is 90° and 0° respectively.

(iii) **Horizontal component of earth's magnetic field :** At a place it is defined as the component of earth's magnetic field along the horizontal in the magnetic meridian.

Its valve is different at different places, (approximately 0.4 gauss or 0.4×10^{-4} tesla).

18. Atomic & Nuclear Physics

Atomic Physics

⇨ Atom is the smallest part of matter which takes part in chemical reactions. Atoms of the same element are similar in mass, size and characteristics. Atom consists of three fundamental particles electron, proton and neutron. All the protons and neutrons are present in the central core of atom called nucleus. Electrons revolve around the nucleus.

⇨ In an atom, electrons and protons are equal in number and have equal and opposite charge. Hence atom is neutral.

Properties of Fundamental Particles

Particle	Mass (Kg)	Charge (Coulomb)	Discoverer
Proton	1.672×10^{-27}	-1.6×10^{-19}	Rutherford
Neutron	1.675×10^{-27}	0	Chadwick
Electron	-9.108×10^{-31}	-1.6×10^{-19}	J.J. Thomson

Note : *Proton was discovered by Golastin and named by Rutherford.*

⇨ Till today, several subatomic particles have been discovered. Some important of them are as follows.

Particle	Mass (Kg)	Charge	Discoverer	
Positron	9.108×10^{-31}	$+1.6 \times 10^{-19}$	Anderson	Antiparticle of electron
Neutrino	0	0	Pauli	
Pi-meson	274 time the mass of electron	Positive and negative both	Yakawa	unstable
Photon	0	0		Velocity equal to that of light

Cathode Rays : If the gas pressure in a discharge tube is 10^{-2} to 10^{-3} mm of Hg and a potential difference of 10^4 volt is applied between the electrode, then a beam of electrons emerges from the cathode which is called cathode rays. Hence cathode rays are beam of high energy electrons. Cathode is an electrode with a negative charge.

Properties of cathode rays :

(i) Cathode rays are invisible and travel in straight line.

(ii) These rays carry negative charge and travel from cathode to anode.

(iii) These rays emerge perpendicular to the cathode surface and are not affected by the position of anode.

(iv) Cathode rays travel with very high velocity (1/10th the velocity of light).

(v) These rays are deflected by electric and magnetic fields.

(vi) These rays can ionise gases.

(vii) These rays heat the material on which they fall.

(viii) They can produce chemical change and thus affect a photographic plate.

(ix) These rays can penetrate through thin metal foils.

(x) The source of emf used in the production of cathode rays is induction coil.

(xi) When they strike a target of heavy metals such as tungsten, they produce x-rays.

(xii) The nature of cathode rays is independent of nature of cathode and the gas in the discharge tube.

Positive or Canal rays :

If perforated cathode is used in a discharge tube, it is observed that a new type of rays are produced from anode moving towards the cathode and passed through the holes of cathode. These rays are positively charged and are called positive rays or canal rays or anode rays. These rays were discovered by *Goldstein*.

Properties of Canal rays :

(i) The positive rays consists of positively charged particles.

(ii) These rays travel in straight line.

(iii) These rays can exert pressure and thus possess kinetic energy.

(iv) These rays are deflected by electric and magnetic fields.

(v) These rays are capable of producing physical and chemical changes.

(vi) These rays can produce ionisation in gases.

Radioactivity

➪ Radioactivity is the sending out of harmful radiation or particles, caused when atomic nuclei breakup spontaneously.

➪ Radioactivity was discovered by *Henry Becquerel, Madame Curie* and *Pierre Curie* for which they jointly win Noble prize.

➪ The nucleus having protons 83 or more are unstable. They emit α, β and γ particles and become stable. The elements of such nucleus are called radioactive elements and the phenomenon of emission of α, β and γ particles is called radioactivity.

➪ γ rays are emitted after the emission of α and β rays.

➪ Robert Pierre and his wife Madame Curie discovered a new radioactive element **radium**.

➪ The rays emitted by radioactivity were first recognised by Rutherford.

➪ The end product of all natural radioactive element after emission of radioactive rays is lead.

Difference between stable and unstable nucleus

S. No.	Stable nucleus	Unstable nucleus
1.	Low atomic number	High atomic number
2.	Low mass number	High mass number
3.	Nucleus of small size	Nucleus of bigger size
4.	$n/p = 1$	$n/p > 1$

Properties of α, β and γ particles

Properties	α	β	γ
Origin	Nucleus	Nucleus	Nucleus
Nature	Positively charged	Negatively charged	Neutral

Composition	He^4	$_1e^0$	Photon
Mass	6.4×10^{-31} kg	9.1×10^{-31} kg	zero
Charge	$+2e$	$-e$	zero
Chemical effect	Affects photographic plate	Affects photographic plate	Affects photo graphic plate
Effect of electric and magnetic field	Deflected	Deflected	No effect
Penetrating power	Minimum	In between the other two	Maximum
Ionising power	Maximum	In between the other two	Minimum
Velocity	Between 1.4×10^7 m/s to 2.2×10^7 m/s	1% to 99% of velocity of light	3×10^8 m/s

⇨ With the emission an α-particle, atomic number is decreased by 2 and mass member is decreased by 4.

⇨ With the emission of a β-particle atomic number is increased by one and mass number does not change.

⇨ The effect on the mass number and atomic number with the emission of α, β and γ rays is decided by **Group-displacement law or Soddy-Fajan Law**.

⇨ Radioactivity is detected by G.M. Counter.

⇨ The time in which half nuclei of the element is decayed is called **half life** of the radioactive substance.

⇨ **Cloud chamber :** Cloud chamber is used to detect the presence and kinetic energy of radioactive particles. It was discovered by C.R.T. Wilson.

⇨ Radioactive carbon-14 is used to measure the age of fossils and plants. (Carbon dating) In this method age is decided by measuring the ratio of $_6C^{12}$ and $_6C^{14}$.

Nuclear Fission and Fusion

Nuclear Fission : The nuclear reaction in which a heavy nucleus splits into two nuclei of nearly equal mass is nuclear fission. The energy released in the nuclear fission is called nuclear energy.

⇨ Nuclear fission was first demonstrated by Strassmann and *O. Hahn*.

They found that when U^{235} nucleus is excited by the capture of a neutron, it splits into two nuclei Ba^{142} & K^{92}.

Chain Reaction: When uranium atom is bombarded with slow neutrons, fission takes place. With the fission of each uranium nucleus, on the average 3 neutrons and large energy is released. These neutrons cause further fission. Clearly a chain of fission of uranium nucleus starts which continues till whole of uranium is exhausted. This is called chain reaction.

⇨ Chain reaction is of the following two types (i) Uncontrolled chain reaction (ii) Controlled chain reaction.

⇨ **Uncontrolled Chain Reaction :** In each fission reaction, three more neutrons are produced. These three neutrons may cause the fission of three other U^{235} nuclei producing 9 neutrons and so on. As a result the number of neutron goes on increasing till the whole of fissionable material is consumed. This chain reaction is called uncontrolled or explosive chain reaction. This reaction proceeds very quickly and a huge amount of energy is liberated in a short time.

Atom bomb : Atom bomb is based on nuclear fission. U^{235} and Pu^{239} are used as fissionable material. This bomb was first used by USA against Japan in second world war (6th August, 1945 at Hiroshima & 9th August, 1945 at Nagashaki).

Controlled Chain Reaction : A fission chain reaction which proceeds slowly without any explosion and in which the energy released can be controlled is known as *controlled reaction*. Actually in this situation only one of the neutrons produced in each fission is able to cause further fission. The rate of reaction remains constant.

Nuclear Reactor or Atomic Pile : Nuclear reactor is an arrangement in which controlled nuclear fission reaction takes place.

⇨ First nuclear reactor was established in Chicago University under the supervision of Prof. Fermi.

⇨ There are several components of nuclear reactor which are as follows :

(i) **Fissionable Fuel :** U^{235} or U^{239} is used.

(ii) **Moderator :** Moderator decreases the energy of neutrons so that they can be further used for fission reaction. Heavy water and graphite are used as moderator.

(iii) **Control rod :** Rods of cadmium or boron are used to absorb the excess neutrons produced in fission of uranium nucleus so that the chain reaction continues to be controlled.

(iv) **Coolant :** A large amount of heat is produced during fission. Coolant absorbs that heat and prevents excessive rise in the temperature. The coolant may be water, heavy water, or a gas like He or CO_2.

Uses of nuclear reactor

(i) To produce electrical energy from the energy released during fission.

(ii) To produce different isotopes which can be used in medical, physical and agriculture science.

Fast Breeder Reactor : A nuclear reactor which can produce more missile fuel than it consumes is called a fast breeder reactor.

Nuclear Fusion : When two or more light nuclei combined together to form a heavier nucleus, tremendous energy is released. This phenomenon is called nuclear fusion. A typical example of nuclear fission is :

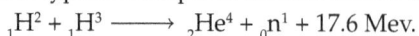

$$_{1}H^{2} + {_{1}H^{3}} \longrightarrow {_{2}He^{4}} + {_{0}n^{1}} + 17.6 \text{ Mev.}$$

⇨ The energy released by sun and other stars is by nuclear fusion.

⇨ For the nuclear fusion, a temperature of the order of 10^8 K is required.

Hydrogen bomb : Hydrogen bomb was made by American scientists in 1952.This is based on nuclear fusion. It is 1000 times more powerful than atom bomb.

Mass Energy Relation : In 1905 Einstein established a relation between mass and energy on the basis of special theory of relativity. According to this relation, mass can be converted into energy and vice versa, according to the relation $E = mc^2$ where c is the velocity of light and E is the energy equivalent of mass m.

⇨ Albert Einstein was an American scientist. He was born in Germany. He was given Nobel Prize of Physics in 1921.

⇨ Sun is continuously emitting energy. Earth is continuously receiving 4×10^{26} joule of energy per second from sun. As a result mass of sun is decreasing at the rate of approximately 4×10^9 kg per second. But mass of sun is so large that it is estimated that the sun will continuously supply energy for next 10^9 years .

19. Electronics

Electronics : Electronics is the branch of physics and technology concerned with the behaviour and movement of electrons.

Diode Valve : Designed by J. A. Fleming in 1904, diode valve consists of two electrodes placed inside an evacuated glass envelope. One electrode is called cathode which is made up of tungsten on which there is a thin layer of barium oxide. When heated, cathode emits electrons. These electron flow towards the other electrode called anode or plate, which is at positive potential. As a result an electric current is established in the circuit.

⇨ The electrons emitted from the cathode are collected in the evaluated space around it. This collection of electrons is called *space charge* which is obviously negative.

⇨ Diode valve acts a rectifier. *Rectifier* is a device which converts alternating voltage (current) into direct voltage (current).

Triode Valve : Designed by Lee de Forest in 1907, triode valve is a modified form of usual diode. It consists of a usual anode-cathode pair and one more electrode called *control grid*.

⇨ Triode valve can be used as amplifier, oscillator, transmitter and detector.

Semi-conductor : Semi-conductor are those materials whose electrical conductivity, at room temperature, lies in between that of insulator and conductor. Germenium and Silicon are two important semi-conductor. In a crystal lattice of semi-conductor, some of the electrons become free from bond formation. At the sites of these electrons a deficiency of electron exists which acts as a virtual positive charge. These virtual positive charges are called holes. Semi-conductors are used in electronics industry.

Semi-conductors are of two types :

(i) **Intrinsic Semi-conductor :** A semi-conductor in an extremely pure form is known as intrinsic semi-conductor.

(ii) **Extrinsic Semi-conductor :** If a measured and small amount of chemical impurity is added to intrinsic semi-conductor, it is called extrinsic semi-conductor or doped semi-conductor. As a result of doping, there is large increase in its conductivity.

⇨ Extrinsic semi-conductor are of two types :

(a) **N type semi-conductor :** An extrinsic semi-conductor in which electrons are majority charge carrier is called N type semi-conductor. Such a semi-conductor is made by doping a pure semi-conductor with pentavalent impurity like Arsenic, Antimony & Phosphorus.

(b) **P type semi-conductor :** An extrinsic semi-conductor in which holes are the majority charge carrier is called a P type semi-conductor. Such a semi conductor is made by doping a pure semi-conductor with trivalent impurity like Gallium, Indium, Boron and Aluminium.

Doping: Adding of chemical impurity to a pure semi conductor is called doping. The amount and type of impurity is closely controlled.

Donor : Pentavalent impurities are called *donor*.

Acceptor : Trivalent impurities are called *acceptor*.

⇨ The electrical conductivity of a semi-conductor increases with the increase in temperature.

Miscellaneous

1. Scientific Instruments

Instrument	Use
Altimeter	Measures altitudes (used in aircraft)
Ammeter	Measures strength of electric current
Anemometer	Measures force and velocity of wind and directions
Audiometer	Measures intensity of sound
Barograph	Continuous recording of atmospheric pressure
Barometer	Measures atmospheric pressure
Binoculars	To view distant objects
Bolometer	To measure heat radiation
Callipers	Measure inner and outer diameters of bodies
Calorimeter	Measures quantities of heat
Cardiogram (ECG)	Traces movements of the heart; recorded on a Cardiograph
Cathetometer	Determines heights, measurement of levels, etc., in scientific experiments
Chronometer	Determines longitude of a vessel at sea

Colorimeter	Compares intensity of colours
Commutator	To change/reverse the direction of electric current; Also used to convert AC into DC
Cryometer	A type of thermometer used to measure very low temperatures, usually close to 0°C
Cyclotron	A charged particle accelerator which can accelerate charged particles to high energies
Dilatometer	Measures changes in volume of substances
Dyanamo	To convert mechanical energy into electrical energy
Dynamometer	Measures electrical power
Electronecephalo graph (EEC)	Records and interprets the electrical waves of the brain (brain waves) recorded on electroence-phalograms
Electrometer	Measures very small but potential difference in electric currents
Electroscope	Detects presence of an electric charge
Electromicroscope	To obtain a magnifying view of very small objects Capable of magnifying up to 20,000 times
Endoscope	To examine internal parts of the body
Fathometer	Measures depth of the ocean
Fluxmeter	Measures magnetic flux
Galvanometer	Measures electric current
Hydrometer	Measures the relative density of liquids
Hygrometer	Measures level of humidity
Hydrophone	Measures sound under water
Hygroscope	Shows the changes in atmospheric humidity
Hypsometer	To determine boiling point of liquids
Kymograph	Graphically records physiological movement. (e.g., blood pressure/heartbeat)
Lactometer	Measures the relative density of milk to determine purity
Machmeter	Determines the speed of an aircraft in terms of the speed of sound
Magnetometer	Compares magnetic movements and fields
Manometer	Measures the pressure of gases
Micrometer	Converts sound waves into electrical vibrations
Microphone	Measures distances/angles

Microscope	To obtain a magnified view of small objects
Nephetometer	Measures the scattering of light by particles suspended in a liquid
Ohmmeter	To measure electrical resistance in ohms
Ondometer	Measures the frequency of electromagnetic waves, especially in the radio-frequency band
Periscope	To view objects above sea level (used in submarines)
Photometer	Compares the luminous intensity of the source of light
Polygraph	Instrument that simultaneously records changes in physiological processes such as heartbeat, blood-pressure and respiration; used as a lie detector
Pyknometer	Determines the density and coefficient of expansion of liquids
Pyrheliometer	Measures components of solar radiation
Pyrometer	Measures very high temperature
Quadrant	Measures altitudes and angles in navigation and astronomy
Radar	To detect the direction and range of an approaching aeroplane by means of radiowaves, (Radio, Angle, Detection and Range)
Radio micrometer	Measures heat radiation
Refractometer	Measures refractive indices
Salinometer	Determines salinity of solutions
Sextant	Used by navigators to find the latitude of a place by measuring the elevation above the horizon of the sun or another star; also used to measure the height of very distant objects
Spectroscope	To observe or record spectra
Spectrometer	Spectroscope equipped with calibrated scale to measure the position of spectral lines (Measurement of refractive indices)
Spherometer	Measures curvature of spherical objects
Sphygmometer	Measures blood pressure
Stereoscope	To view two-dimensional pictures
Stethoscope	Used by doctors to hear and analyze heart and lung sounds
Stroboscope	To view rapidly moving objects

Tachometer	To determine speed, especially the rotational speed of a shaft (used in aeroplanes and motor-boats)
Tacheometer	A theodolite adapted to measure distances, elevations and bearings during survey
Tangent Galvanometer	Measures the strength of direct current
Telemeter	Records physical happenings at a distant place
Teleprinter	Receives and sends typed messages from one place to another
Telescope	To view distant objects in space
Thermometer	Measures Temperature
Thermostat	Regulates temperature at a particular point
Tonometer	To measure the pitch of a sound
Transponder	To receive a signal and transmit a reply immediately
Udometer	Rain gauge
Ultrasonoscope	To measure and use ultrasonic sound (beyond hearing); use to make a Ecogram to detect brain tumours, heart defects and abnormal growth
Venturimeter	To measure the rate of flow of liquids
Vernier	Measures small sub-division of scale
Viscometer	Measures the viscosity of liquid
Voltmeter	To measure electric potential difference between two points
Wattmeter	To measure the power of an electric circuit
Wavemeter	To measure the wavelength of a radiowave

2. Inventions

Invention	Inventor	Country	Year
Adding machine	Pascal	France	1642
Aeroplane	Wright brothers	USA	1903
Balloon	Jacques and Joseph Montgolfier	France	1783
Ball-point pen	C. Biro	Hungary	1938
Barometer	E. Torricelli	Italy	1644
Bicycle	K. Macmillan	Scotland	1839
Bicycle Tyre	J.B. Dunlop	Scotland	1888

Calculating machine	Pascal	France	1642
Centrigrade scale	A. Celsius	France	1742
Cinematograph	Thomas Alva Edison	USA	1891
Computer	Charles Babbage	Britain	1834
Cine camera	Friese-Greene	Britain	1889
Cinema	A.L. and J.L. Lumiere	France	1895
Clock (machanical)	Hsing and Ling-Tsan	China	1725
Clock (pendulum)	C. Hugyens	Netherlands	1657
Diesel engine	Rudolf Diesel	Germany	1892
Dynamite	Alfred Nobel	Sweden	1867
Dynamo	Michael Faraday	England	1831
Electric iron	H.W. Seeley	USA	1882
Electric lamp	Thomas Alva Edison	USA	1879
Electromagnet	W. Sturgeon	England	1824
Evolution (theory)	Charles Darwin	England	1858
Film (with sound)	Dr Lee de Forest	USA	1923
Fountain Pen	LE. Waterman	USA	1884
Gas lighting	William Murdoch	Scotland	1794
Gramophone	T.A. Edison	USA	1878
Jet Engine	Sir Frank Whittle	England	1937
Lift	E.G. Otis	USA	1852
Locomotive	Richard Trevithick	England	1804
Machine gun	Richard Gatling	USA	1861
Match (safety)	J.E. Lurdstrom	Sweden	1855
Microphone	David Hughes	USA	1878
Microscope	Z. Jansen	Netherlands	1590
Motor car (petrol)	Karl Benz	Germany	1885
Motorcycle	Edward Butler	England	1884
Neon-lamp	G. Claude	France	1915
Nylon	Dr W.H. Carothers	USA	1937
Photography (paper)	W.H. Fox Tablot	England	1835
Printing press	J.Gutenberg	Germany	1455
Radar	Dr A.H. Taylor and L.C. Young	USA	1922
Radium	Marie and Pierre Curie	France	1898

Radio	G. Marconi	England	1901
Rayon	American Viscose Co.	USA	1910
Razor (safety)	K.G. Gillette	USA	1895
Razor (electric)	Col. J. Schick	USA	1931
Refrigerator	J. Harrison and A. Catlin	Britain	1834
Revolver	Samuel Colt	USA	1835
Rubber (vulcanized)	Charles Goodyear	USA	1841
Rubber (waterproof)	Charles Macintosh	Scotland	1819
Safety lamp	Sir Humphrey Davy	England	1816
Safety pin	William Hurst	USA	1849
Sewing machine	B. Thimmonnier	France	1830
Scooter	G. Bradshaw	England	1919
Ship (steam)	J.C. Perier	France	1775
Ship (turbine)	Sir Charles Parsons	Britain	1894
Shorthand (modem)	Sir Issac Pitman	Britain	1837
Spinning frame	Sir Richard Arkwight	England	1769
Spinning jenny	James Hargreaves	England	1764
Steam engine (piston)	Thomas Newcome	Britain	1712
Steam engine (condenser)	James Watt	Scotland	1765
Steel production	Henry Bessemer	England	1855
Stainless Steel	Harry Brearley	England	1913
Tank	Sir Ernest Swington	England	1914
Telegraph code	Samuel F.B. Morse	USA	1837
Telephone	Alexander Graham Bell	USA	1876
Telescope	Hans Lippershey	Netherlands	1608
Television	John Logie Bared	Scotland	1926
Terylene	J. Whinfield and H. Dickson	England	1941
Thermometer	Galileo Galilei	Italy	1593
Tractor	J. Froelich	USA	1892
Transistor	Bardeen, Shockley	USA & UK	1949
Typewriter	C. Sholes	USA	1868
Valve of radio	Sir J.A. Fleming	Britain	1904

Watch	A.L. Breguet	France	1791
X-ray	Wilhelm Roentgen	Germany	1895
Zip fastener	W.L. Judson	USA	1891

3. Important Discoveries in Physics

Discovery	Scientist	Year
Laws of motion	Newton	1687
Law of electrostatic attraction	Coulomb	1779
Atom	John Dalton	1808
Photography (On metal)	J. Neepse	1826
Law of Electric resistance	G.S.Ohm	1827
Law of floatation	Archemedes	1827
Electromagnetic Induction	Michael Faraday	1831
Photography (On paper)	W.Fox Talbot	1835
Dynamite	Alfred Nobel	1867
Periodic table	Mandeleev	1888
X-Rays	Roentgen	1895
Radioactivity	Henry Becquerel	1896
Electron	J. J. Thomson	1897
Radium	Madam Curie	1898
Quantum theory	Max Plank	1900
Wireless Telegram	Marconi	1901
Diode Bulb	Sir J. S. Fleming	1904
Photo electric effect	Albert Einstein	1905
Principle of Relativity	Albert Einstein	1905
Triode Bulb	Lee de Forest	1906
Atomic Structure	Neil Bohr & Rutherford	1913
Proton	Rutherford	1919
Raman Effect	C.V. Raman	1928
Neutron	James Chadwick	1932
Nuclear Reactor	Amico Fermi	1942
Law of electrolytic dissociation	Faraday	—
Thermionic emission	Edison	—

4. S.l. Units of Physical Quantity

Quantity	SI	Symbol
Length	meter	m
Mass	kilogram	kg
Time	second	s
Work and Energy	joule	J
Electric current	ampere	A
Temperature	kelvin	K
Intensity of flame	candela	cd
Angle	radian	rad
Solid angle	steredian	sr
Force	newton	N
Area	square meter	m^2
Volume	Cubic meter	m^3
Speed	meter per second	ms^{-1}
Angle velocity	radian per second	$rad\ s^{-1}$
Frequency	Hertz	Hz
Moment of inertia	kilogram Square meter	kgm^2
Momentum	kilogram meter per second	$Kg\ ms^{-1}$
impulse	newton second	Ns
Angular momentum	kilogram square meter per second	Kgm^2s^{-1}
Pressure	pascal	Pa
Power	watt	W
Surface tension	newton per meter	Nm^{-1}
Viscosity	newton second per square m	$N.s.m^{-2}$
Thermal conductivity	watt per meter per degree celcius	$wm^{-1}C^{-1}$
Specific heat capacity	joule per kilogram per Kelvin	$Jkg^{-1}\ K^{-1}$
Electric charge	coulomb	c
Potential difference	volt	v
Electric resistance	ohm	
Electrical capacity	farad	F

Magnetic induction	henry	H
Magnetic Flux	weber	Wb
Luminous Flux or photometric power	lumen	lm
Intensity of illumination	lux	lx
Wavelength	Angstrom	A°
Astronomical distance	light year	ly

5. Conversion of Units
(From One System to Another System)

1 Inch	2.54 centimeter	1 grain	64.8 miligram
1 Feet	0.3 meter	1 dram	1.77 gm
1 Yard	0.91 meter	1 ounce	28.35 gm
1 Mile	1.60 kilometer	1 pound	0.4537 kilogram
1 Fathom	1.8 meter	1 dyne	10^{-5} Newton
1 Chain	20.11 meter	1 poundal	0.1383 Newton
1 Nautical mile	1.85 kilometer	1 erg	10^{-7} Joule
1 Angstrom	10^{-10} meter	1 horse power	747 Watt
1 Square inch	6.45 sq. centimeter	1 fathom	6 feet
1 Square feet	0.09 square meter	1 mile	8 furlong
1 Square yard	0.83 square meter	1 mile	5280 feet
1 Acre	10^4 sq. meter	1 nautical mile	6080 feet
1 Square mile	2.58 sq. kilometer	1 feet	12 inch
1 Cubic inch	16.38 cubic centimeter	1 yard	3 feet
1 Cubic feet	0.028 cubic meter	37° centigrade	98.6° Fahrenheit
1 Cubic yard	0.7 quebec meter	50° centigrade	122 Fahrenheit
1 Litre	1000 cubic centimeter	–40° Fahrenheit	–40° Centigrade
1 Pint	0.56 litre	32° Fahrenheit	0° Centigrade

Chemistry

1. Introduction

Chemistry is the branch of science which deals with the composition of matter and also the Physical and Chemical characteristics associated with the different material objects.

A French chemist, *Lavoisier (1743-1793)* is regarded as father of modern chemistry.

Branches of Chemistry

⇨ *Organic Chemistry*: This branch of chemistry deals with the study of the organic matter. The substances that primarily consist of carbon and hydrogen are termed as organic. It is the study of the structure, composition and the chemical properties of organic compounds and the chemical reactions that are a part of making organic chemical compounds.

➭ *Inorganic Chemistry*: this is that branch which studies the elements, their compounds and their properties.

➭ *Physical Chemistry*: this branch studies physical phenomena. The theories of physics are applied to atomic and subatomic particles.

➭ *Biochemistry*: It deals with the structure and behaviour of the components of cells and the chemical processes in living beings.

➭ *Nuclear Chemistry*: it studies radioactivity. It deals with the nuclear properties of and the chemical processes in radioactive substances.

1. Substance and its nature : Anything that occupies space, possesses mass and can be felt by any one or more of our senses is called matter.

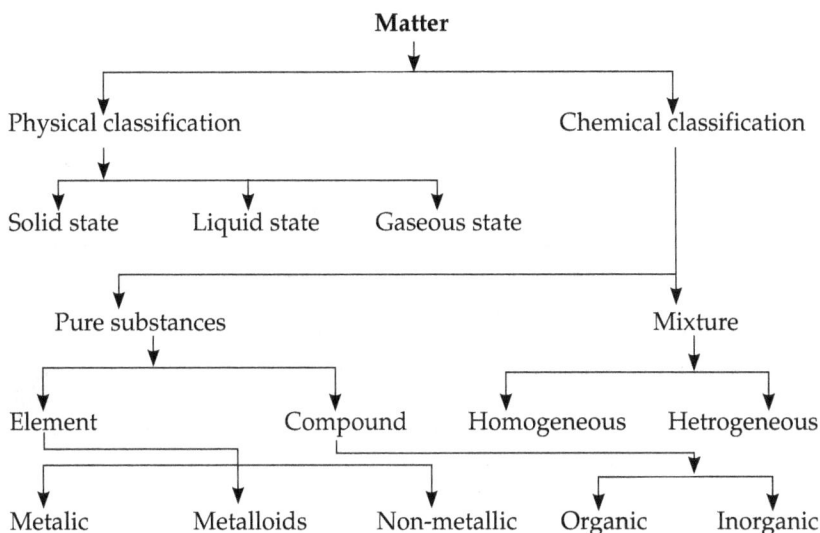

Solid State : A solid possesses definite shape and definite volume which means that it can not be compressed on applying pressure. Solids are generally hard and rigid. *Example*— metals, wood, bricks, copper etc.

Liquid State : A liquid possesses definite volume but no definite shape. This means that the liquid can take up the shape of container in which it is placed. *Example*— water, milk, oil, alcohol etc.

Gaseous State : A gas does not have either a definite volume or definite shape. It can be compressed to large extent on applying pressure and also takes the shape of the container where it is enclosed. *Examples*— Air, Oxygen, Nitrogen, Ammonia, Carbondioxide etc.

Solid state $\xrightleftharpoons[\text{Cool}]{\text{Heat}}$ Liquid state $\xrightleftharpoons[\text{Cool}]{\text{Heat}}$ Vapour state

Water exists in three different states.

Ice $\rightleftharpoons$ Water $\rightleftharpoons$ Vapour
(Solid)   (Liquid)   (Gas)

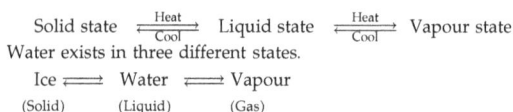

Pure Substances : A single substance (or matter) which can not be separated into other kinds of matter by any physical process is called pure substance.

Pure substances have been classified as elements and compounds.

Elements : The simplest form of a pure substance which can neither be broken into nor built from simpler substances by ordinary physical and chemical methods is called element.

Elements are further classified into three types (i) Metals (ii) Non-metals and (iii) Metalloids.

Metals : Metals are solids (exception mercury which is liquid at room temperature) are normally hard. They have lustre, high *mp* and *bp* and also good conductor of electricity and heat. The conductivity of metal decreases with increase in temperature due to vibration of positive ions at their Lattice points. *Examples* — Iron, Copper, Silver, Gold, Aluminium, Zinc etc.

Non-metals : Non-metals are the elements with properties opposite to those of the metals. They are found in all states of matter. They do not possess lustre (exception-iodine). They are poor conductors of electricity (exception graphite) and they are not malleable and ductile. *Examples* — Hydrogen, Carbon, Oxygen, Nitrogen, Sulphur, Phosphorous etc.

Metalloids : Metalloids are the elements which have common properties of both metals and non-metals. *Examples*— Arsenic, Antimony, Bismuth etc.

Compounds : Compounds are pure substances that are composed of two or more different elements in fixed proportion by mass.The properties of a compound are entirely different from those of the elements from which it is made. *Example*— Water, Sugar, Salt, chloroform, Alcohol, Ether etc.

Compounds are classified into two types

(i) Organic compounds   (ii) Inorganic compounds,

Organic Compounds : The Compounds obtained from living sources are called organic compounds. The term organic is now applied to hydrocarbons and their derivatives. *Examples*— Carbohydrates, Proteins, Oils, Fats etc.

Inorganic Compounds : The Compounds obtained from non-living sources such as rocks and minerals are called inorganic compounds. *Examples*— Common Salt, Marble, Washing Soda etc.

Mixtures : A material obtained by mixing two or more substances in any indefinite proportion is called a mixture. The properties of the components in a mixture remain unchanged. *Example*— Milk, Sea water, Petrol, Paint, Glass, Cement, Wood etc.

There are two types of mixture—

(1) Homogeneous mixture   (2) Heterogeneous mixture.

1. **Homogeneous mixture :** A mixture is said to be homogeneous if it has a uniform composition through out and there are no visible boundaries of separation between constituents. More over, the constituents can not be seen even by a microscope. *Examples* — Common salt dissolved in water, sugar dissolved in water, iodine dissolved in CCl_4, benzene in toluene and methyl alcohol in water.
2. **Heterogeneous mixture :** A mixture is said to be heterogeneous if it does not have a uniform composition throughout and has visible boundaries of separation between the various constituents. The different constituents of the heterogeneous mixture can be seen even with naked eye. *Example* — A mixture of Sulphur & Sand, A mixture of Iron filings & Sand etc.

Separation of Mixture : Some methods of separation of mixtures are given below:

1. **Sublimation :** In this process, a solid substance passes direct into its vapours on application of heat. The vapours when cooled, give back the original substance. This method can be used for the substances which are sublime in their separation from non-sublimate materials. Examples of sublimes are Naphthalene, Iodine, Ammonium Chloride etc.

2. **Filtration :** This is a process for quick and complete removal of suspended solid particles from a liquid, by passing the suspension through a filter paper. *Examples*— (i) removed of solid particles from the engine oil in car engine. (ii) filtration of tea from tea leaves in the preparation of tea etc.

3. **Evaporation :** If a solution of solid substance in a liquid is heated, the liquid gets converted into its vapours and slowly goes off completely. This process is called evaporation. *Example*— (i) Evaporation of water in summer from Ponds, wells & lakes. (ii) Preparation of common salt from sea water by evaporation of water.

4. **Crystallization :** This method is mostly used for separation and purification of solid substances. In this process, the impure solid or mixture is heated with suitable solvent (*e.g.* alcohol, water, acetone, chloroform) to its boiling point and the hot solution is filtered. The clear filtrate is cooled slowly to room temperature, when pure solid crystallizes out. This is separated by filtration and dried.

For the separation of more complex mixtures, fractional crystallization is used, in which the components of the mixtures crystallize out at different interval of time.

5. **Distillation :** It is a process of converting a liquid into its vapour by heating and then condensing the vapour again into the same liquid by cooling. Thus, distillation involves vaporisation and condensation both

Distillation = Vaporisation + Condensation

This method is employed to separate the liquids which have different boiling points or a liquid from non-volatile solid or solids either in solution or suspension. *Example*— A mixture of copper sulphate and water or a mixture of water (B.P 100°C) and methyl alcohol (B.P 45°C) can be separated by this method.

6. Fractional distillation : This prucess is similar to the distillation process except that a fractionating column is used to separate two or more volatile liquid which have different boiling points. *Example*— (i) Methyl alcohol (bp = 338 K) and acetone (bp = 329 K) can be separated by fractional distillation process. (ii) Separation of petrol, diesel oil, kerosene oil, heavy oil etc from crude petroleum. (iii) Separation of oxygen, nitrogen inert gasses and carbon dioxide from liquid air etc.

7. Chromatography : The name chromatography is derived from Latin word 'Chroma' meaning colour. The technique of chromatography is based on the difference in the rates at which the components of a mixture are absorbed in the suitable absorbent.

There are many types of chromatography.

(a) Column (absorption) chromatography

(b) Thin layer chromatography

(c) Paper- chromatography

(d) High pressure liquid chromatography

(e) In-exchange chromatography

(f) Gas chromatography

8. Sedimentation and Decantation : This method is used when one component is a liquid and other is an insoluble. Insoluble solid, heavier than liquid. i.e, mud and water.

If muddy water is allowed to stand undisturbed for sometime in a beaker, the particles of earth (clay and sand) settle at the bottom. This process is called sedimentation. The clear liquid at the top can be gently transferred into another beaker. This process is known as decantation.

Concept of change in state : (a) Melting Point : The temperature at which solid and the liquid forms of the substance exist at equilibrium or both forms have same vapour pressure is called melting point.

(b) Boiling point : The temperature at which the vapour pressure of the liquid is equal to atmospheric pressure is called boiling point.

Liquid	Water	Ethanol	Chloroform	Acetone
B.P.	373 K	349 K	334 K	329 K

(c) Freezing Point : The temperature at which the vapour pressure of its liquid is equal to the vapour pressure of the corresponding solid is called *freezing point.*

(d) Evaporation : The process of conversion of a liquid into its vapours at room temperature is called evaporation. Evaporation causes cooling. Actually, during evaporation, the molecules having higher kinetic energy escape from the surface of the liquid. Therefore, average kinetic energy of the rest of the molecules decreases. Therefore cooling takes place during

evaporation because of temperature of liquid is directly proportional to average kinetic Energy. Evaporation is affected by following factors,

(i) Nature of liquid (ii) Temperature (iii) Surface area

(e) Vapour pressure: The pressure exerted by the vapours of liquid in equilibrium with liquid at a given temperature is called vapour pressure. Vapour pressure depends upon—(i) its nature and (ii) temperature.

Higher the vapour pressure of a particular liquid lesser will be the magnitude of intermolecular forces present in molecules. Vapour pressure of a liquid increases with increase in temperature.

2. Atomic Structure

Atom : The smallest particle of an element is called an atom. An atom can take part in chemical combination and does not occur free in nature. The atom of the hydrogen is the smallest and lightest. *Example* — Na, K, Ca, H etc.

Molecule: A molecule is the smallest particle of an element or compound that can have a stable and independent existence. Example—O_2, N_2, Cl_2, P_4, S_8 etc.

Mole : A mole is a collection of 6.023×10^{23} particles. It means that

1 mole = 6.023×10^{23}

1 mole atom = 6.023×10^{23} atoms

1 mole molecule = 6.023×10^{23} molecules

1 mole ion = 6.023×10^{23} ions

1 mole mango = 6.023×10^{23} mangoes

1 mole Apple = 6.023×10^{23} apples

Avogadro's Number : The number 6.023×10^{23} is called Avogadro's Number.

Atomic Mass : It is the ratio of mass of one atom of the element to 1/12th part of the mass of one atom of carbon — 12.

$$\text{Atomic mass of an element} = \frac{\text{Mass of one atom of the element}}{\frac{1}{12} \times \text{mass of one atom of carbon} - 12}$$

Actual mass of 1 atom of an element = atomic mass in amu $\times$ 1.66×10^{-24} g

Molecular mass : It indicates how many times one molecule of a substance is heavier in comparison to 1/12th mass of one atom of Carbon–12.

Constituents of an atom: Fundamental particles of an atom are Electron, Proton & Neutron.

Electron :

(i) Electron had been discovered by *J. J. Thomson.*

(ii) The name of electron was given by *Stoney.*

(iii) Charge on an electron $\Big\langle$ relative — – 1 unit

absolute — -1.6×10^{-19} coulomb

or $- 4.8 \times 10^{-10}$ e.s.u

(iv) Mass of an electron $\Big\langle$ relative — 0.000543 amu

absolute — 9.1×10^{-28} g

(v) $\dfrac{\text{charge}}{\text{mass}}\left(\dfrac{e}{m}\right)$ ratio of electron $= - 1.76 \times 10^8 \ \dfrac{C}{g}$

(vi) An electron was obtained from Cathode rays experimental.

Proton :

(i) A proton had been discovered by *Goldstein*.

(ii) A proton was named by *Rutherford*.

(iii) Charge on proton $\Big\langle$ relative — + 1 unit

absolute — $+ 1.6 \times 10^{-19}$ C

or $+ 4.8 \times 10^{-10}$ e.s.u.

(iv) Mass of proton $\Big\langle$ relative — 1.00763 amu

absolute — 1.673×10^{-24} g

(v) $\dfrac{\text{charge}}{\text{mass}}$ ratio of proton $= 9.58 \times 10^4 \ \dfrac{C}{g}$

(vi) An proton was obtained from anode rays experiment.

Neutron :

(i) A neutron had been discovered by *James Chadwick*.

(ii) Charge on neutron—zero

(iii) Mass of proton $\Big\langle$ relative — 1.00863 amu

absolute — 1.675×10^{-24} g

(iv) $\dfrac{\text{charge}}{\text{mass}}$ ratio of neutron = zero

(v) A neutron was obtained from radioactivity phenomenon.

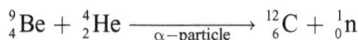

$$_4^9\text{Be} + \,_2^4\text{He} \xrightarrow[\alpha-\text{particle}]{} \,_6^{12}\text{C} + \,_0^1\text{n}$$

Atomic number (Z) : The number of proton or electron in an atom of the element is called atomic number. It is denoted by Z.

Z = e = p where, e = no. of electrons and p = no. of protons.

Mass number (A) : The sum of number or protons and neutrons in an atom of the element is called mass number. It is denoted by A.

$A = p + n$, where, p = no. of protons and n = no. of neutrons

Let, $_{11}^{23}\text{Na}$,

In Na, $Z = 11$, $A = 23$ and,

$\qquad e = 11$, $p = 11$

$\therefore \qquad n = A - p = 23 - 11 = 12$

Isotopes : These are atoms of the elements having the same atomic number but different mass number.

Isotopes of Carbon $- \, _{6}^{12}\text{C}, \, _{6}^{13}\text{C}, \, _{6}^{14}\text{C}$

Isobars : These are atoms of the elements having the same mass number but different atomic numbers. e.g.

$_{18}^{40}\text{Ar}, \, _{19}^{40}\text{K}, \, _{20}^{40}\text{Ca}$

Isotones : These are atoms of different elements having the same number of neutrons.

$_{6}^{14}\text{C}, \, _{7}^{15}\text{K}, \, _{8}^{16}\text{O}$

Isoelectronic : These are atoms/molecules/ions containing the same number of electrons.

(i) O^{2-}, F^-, Ne, Na^+, Mg^{2+} (ii) CN^-, N_2, O_2^{2+} etc.

'Th ' d

Thomson's model of an atom . According to Thomson, an atom is treated as sphere of radius 10^{-8} cm in which positively charged particles are uninformally distributed and negatively charged electrons and embedded through them. This is also called Plum-Pudding model of an atom or water-melon model of an atom.

Rutherford's model of an atom: On the basis of scattering experiment, Rutherford proposed a model of the atom which is known as nuclear atomic model.

According to this model,

(i) An atom consists of a heavy positively charged nucleus where all protons and neutrons are present. Protons & neutrons are collectively called nucleons. Almost whole mass of the atom is contributed by these nucleons.

(ii) Radius of a nucleus = 10^{-13} cm

Radius of an atom = 10^{-8} cm

Radius of an atom = 10^5 times of the radius of the nucleons.

(iii) $\dfrac{\text{Volume of atom}}{\text{Volume of a nucleus}} = \dfrac{\frac{4}{3}\pi(10^{-8})^3}{\frac{4}{3}\pi(10^{-13})^3} = \dfrac{10^{-24}}{10^{-39}} = 10^{15}$

So, volume of an atom is 10^{15} times heavier than volume of a nucleus.

(iv) Electrons revolve around the nucleus in closed orbits with high speed. This model is similar to the solar system, the nucleus representing the sun and revolving electrons as planets. The electrons are therefore, generally referred as planetary electrons.

Spectrum: When white light is allowed to pass through a prism, it splits into several colours. These seven coloured band is called spectrum.

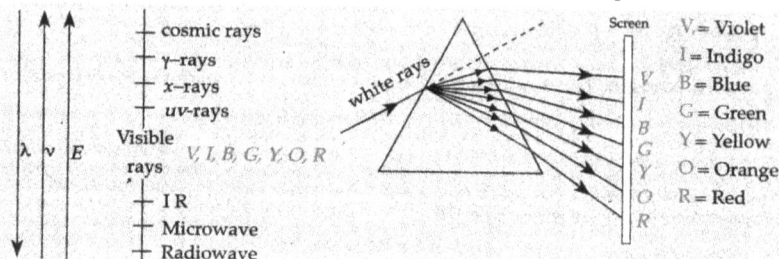

Zeeman's effect : When spectral lines obtained from atomic spectra is placed in a magnetic field, they are splitted into number of fine lines, this is called *Zeeman's effect*.

Stark's effect : When spectral lines obtained from atomic spectra is placed in electric field, they are splitted into number of fine lines this is called Stark's effect.

Thomson's model	Plum pudding model (watermelon model)
Rutherford's model	Nuclear theory
Bohr's model	Concept of quantization of energy
Planck's Quantum theory	Photon & quanta
Sommerfeld's model	Orbital : elliptical & spherical
de-Broglie's equation	Dual nature of electron
Heisenberg's Uncertainty principle	Exact position & momentum can not be determined simultaneously
Schrodinger's wave equation	wave nature of electron

3. Periodic Classification of Elements

Father of periodic table—Mendeleev.

The arrangement of the known elements in certain groups in such a way so that the elements with similar properties are grouped together is known as classification of elements.

Genesis of Periodic Classification :

1. **Lavoisier** classified the elements into metals and non-metals.
2. **Dobereinier's Triads :** In 1829, Dobereiner, a German chemist arranged certain elements with similar properties in groups of

three in such a way that the atomic mass of the middle element was nearly the same as the average atomic masses of the first and third elements.

Triad	Lithium	Sodium	Potassium
Atomic mass	7	23	39

atomic mass of sodium = $\dfrac{39+7}{2} = \dfrac{46}{2} = 23$

But only few elements could be covered under triads.

3. **Newland's law of octaves :** In 1866, John Newlands, An English Chemist proposed the law of octaves by stating that, *When elements are arranged in order to increasing atomic masses, evezy eighth element has properties similar to the first, just like musical notes.*

But this generalization was also rejected because it could not be extended to the elements with atomic mass more than 40.

4. **Lother's–Mayer's atomic volume curve :** In 1869 Lother mayer plotted a graph between atomic volume of the elements and their atomic mass and he pointed that the elements with similar properties occupy similar position in the curve.

5. **Mendeleev's periodic law :** The physical and chemical properties of the elemen s are the periodic function of their atomic masses.

Mendeleev's arranged the elements known at that time in increasing order of atomic masses and this arrangement was periodic table.

In periodic table :

Horizontal line is called periods.

Vertical line is called group.

In Mendeleev's periodic table:

Period-7

Group- 9 (I, II, III, IV, V, VI, VII, VIII, Zero)

6. **Modern Periodic law :** Modern periodic law was given by Moseley.

According to Moseley : "The physical and chemical properties of the elements are the periodic function of their atomic numbers."

In modern periodic table :

Period—7   Group—18

Modern periodic table are classified as :

(i) s–block   (ii) p–block

(iii) d–block   (iv) f–block

    s-block : Alkali & Alkaline earth metals.

    p-block : Chalcogen, Picogens, Halogens and inert gases.

    d-block : Transition elements.

    f-block : Inner transition elements.

Periodic properties :

(i) **Atomic radii :** The distance from the centre of the nucleus to the outermost shell containing electrons called atomic radius.

It is not possible to measure the absolute value of atomic radius of an element. However, it may be expressed in three different form covalent radii, metallic radii, Van der wall radii.

Van der wall radii > metallic radii > covalent radii.

(ii) **Ionic radii :** The effective distance from the centre of nucleus of the ion upto which it exerts its influence on the electron cloud is called ionic radii.

Anionic radii > atomic radii > cationic radii

(iii) **Ionization Potential (I.P.) :** The amount of energy required to remove an electron from isolated gaseous atom is called Ionization Potential (I.P.) or Ionization Energy (I.E.)

A (g) $- e +$ Energy required (I.P.) $\rightarrow A^+$ (g)

(iv) **Electron affinity (E_a) :** The energy released during addition of an extra electron in isolated gaseous atom is called electron Affinity.

A (g) $+ e \rightarrow A^-$ (g) $+$ Energy released

Chlorine (Cl) has highest E_a value.

(v) **Electronegativity (E_n) :** The relative electron attracting tendency of its atom for a shared pair of electrons in a chemical bond is called electronegativity.

F is the most electronegative atom

$$E_n = \frac{IP + E_a}{5.6}$$

E_n value > 1.7 (ionic compound)

E_n value < 1.7 (polar covalent compound)

E_n value = 0 (nonpolar compound)

(vi) **Lattice Energy :** The amount of energy released during formation of one mole of ionic compound from its constituent ions is called Lattice energy.

(vii) **Hydration Energy:** The amount of energy released during dissolution of one mole of compound into water, is called hydration energy.

If hydration nergy > Lattice energy, then compound is soluble in water and if hydration energy < Lattice energy, then compound is insoluble in water.

4. Chemical Bonding

The force that holds together the different atoms in a molecule is called *chemical bond*. There are many types of chemical bond.

1. **Ionic bond or (Electrovalent bond)** : A bond formed by the complete transfer of one or more electrons from one atom to other atom is called ionic bond. *Example—*

(a) Formation of NaCl :

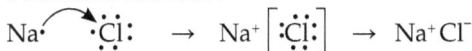

$$Na \cdot \quad \cdot \overset{\cdot\cdot}{\underset{\cdot\cdot}{Cl}}: \quad \rightarrow \quad Na^+ \left[:\overset{\cdot\cdot}{\underset{\cdot\cdot}{Cl}}: \right] \quad \rightarrow \quad Na^+ Cl^-$$

Condition of ionic bond : I. Ionization energy of metal should be low. II. Electron affinity of non-metal should be high.

Properties of ionic compounds :

(a) Ionic compounds have high melting point & boiling point.

(b) Ionic compounds are good conductor of electricity in molten state or in water.

(c) Ionic compounds are bad conductor of electricity in solid state.

(d) Ionic compounds are soluble in water.

(e) Ionic cqmpounds are insoluble in non-polar covalent like Benzene, Carbon tetrachloride etc.

Covalent bond : A bond formed between two same or different atoms by mutual contribution and sharing of electrons is called covalent bond. *Example—*

(a) H_2 molecule :

$$(H \cdot \! \cdot \! H) \quad \rightarrow \quad H-H$$

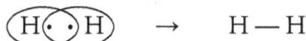

(b) Cl_2 molecule :

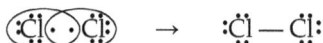

$$(\overset{\cdot\cdot}{\underset{\cdot\cdot}{Cl}} \! \cdot \! \cdot \! \overset{\cdot\cdot}{\underset{\cdot\cdot}{Cl}}) \quad \rightarrow \quad :\overset{\cdot\cdot}{Cl}-\overset{\cdot\cdot}{Cl}:$$

(c) CH_4 molecule :

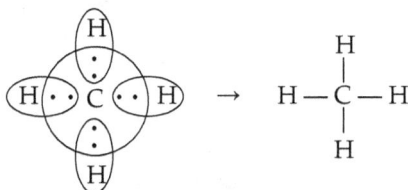

$$\rightarrow \quad H-\underset{\underset{H}{|}}{\overset{\overset{H}{|}}{C}}-H$$

Properties of covalent compounds:

(a) Covalent compounds have high m.p. & b.p.

(b) They are generally bad conductor of electricity (exception graphite)

(c) They are generally insoluble in water.

(d) They are generally soluble in organic solvent like benzene, acetone, chloroform etc.

(e) Covalent bonds are directional.

Co-ordinate bond (or Dative bond) : Co-ordinate bond is a special type of covalent bond in which one atom donates electrons to other atom. The bonding between donor to acceptor atom is called co-ordinate bond. It is denoted by →. *Example—*

SO_2 $\ddot{O}(::)\ddot{S}:$ → $:\ddot{O}:$ → O = S → O

Sigma bond (σ-bond) : A bond formed by the linear overlapping of atomic orbitals is called sigma bond. Since, the extent of overlapping of atomic orbitals in σ-bond in large. Hence σ-bond is a strong bond.

Pi-bond (π-bond) : A bond formed by the sidewise (or lateral overlapping of atomic orbitals is called π-bond. Since, in this case, extent of overlapping of atomic orbitals is lesser than σ-bond. So, π-bond is a weak bond.

$$H \underset{\sigma}{\longrightarrow} H ; \quad O \underset{\sigma}{\overset{\pi}{=\!=}} O ; \quad N \underset{\overset{\sigma}{\underline{\pi}}}{\overset{\pi}{\equiv}} N$$

Bond energy : The amount of energy required to break one mole bonds of a particular type between the atoms in the gaseous state of a substance is called bond energy. The bond energy depends upon the following factors.

(i) Size of atom   (ii) Multiplicity of bonds.

Greater the size of atoms, Lesser will be bond energy.

Greater the bond multiplicity more will be bond energy.

Bond energy : Single bond < double bond < triple bond

Bond length : The average equilibrium distance between the centres of the two bonded atoms is called bond length. The bond length is influenced by the following factors —

(i) Size of atoms   (ii) Multiplicity of bonds

Greater the size of atoms, greater will be bond length.

Greater the multiplicity of bonds, lesser will be bond length.

Hydrogen bond : When hydrogen atom is present between two most electronegative atoms (N, O, F) then it is bonded to one by a covalent bond and to other by a weak force of attraction which is called hydrogen bond. etc. It is denoted by .... *Example—*

(i) $(HF)_n$

     H — F ·········   H — F ·········   H — F ·········   H — F

(ii) $(H_2O)_n$

     ········· H — O ·········   H — O ·········   H — O ·········
                 | | |
                 H   H   H

(iii)

O —Nitrophenol

There are two type of hydrogen bonding

(i) Intermolecular hydrogen bond.

(ii) Intramolecular hydrogen bond.

Intermolecular hydrogen bond arises when hydrogen bonding occurs between two or more molecules. In this case m.p. & b.p. of compound increases due to molecular association.

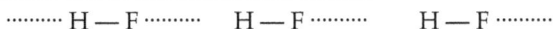

·········· H — F ·········· H — F ·········· H — F ··········

When hydrogen bonding occurs within a molecule then it is called intramolecular hydrogen bonding. Due to cyclisation m.p. & b.p. of the compound decreases in this case.

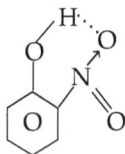

Due to intermolecular hydrogen bonding between alcohol and water alcohol is soluble in water.

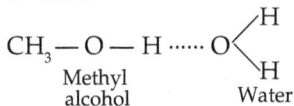

$$CH_3 - O - H \cdots\cdots O \underset{H}{\overset{H}{<}}$$

Methyl alcohol   Water

5. Oxidation and Reduction

Oxidation (old concept) : Oxidation is a process which involves either of the following:

(i) addition of oxygen

(ii) removal of hydrogen

(iii) addition of electro negative element or group

(iv) removal of electro positive element or group.

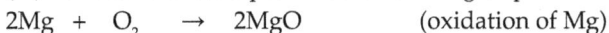

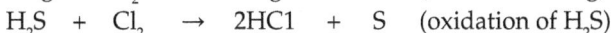

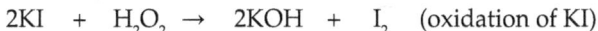

$2Mg + O_2$	$\rightarrow$	$2MgO$	(oxidation of Mg)
$H_2S + Cl_2$	$\rightarrow$	$2HCl + S$	(oxidation of H_2S)
$Fe + S$	$\rightarrow$	FeS	(oxidation of Fe)
$2KI + H_2O_2$	$\rightarrow$	$2KOH + I_2$	(oxidation of KI)

Reduction (old concept) : Reduction is a process which involves either of the following—

(i) addition of hydrogen

(ii) removal of oxygen

(iii) addition of electro positive element or group.

(iv) removal of electronegative element or group.

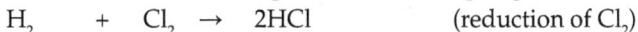

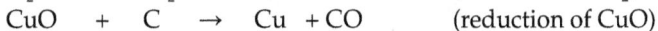

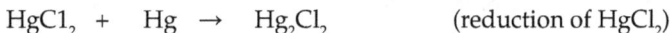

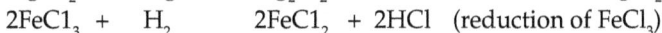

$H_2 + Cl_2$	$\rightarrow$	$2HCl$	(reduction of Cl_2)
$CuO + C$	$\rightarrow$	$Cu + CO$	(reduction of CuO)
$HgCl_2 + Hg$	$\rightarrow$	Hg_2Cl_2	(reduction of $HgCl_2$)
$2FeCl_3 + H_2$		$2FeCl_2 + 2HCl$	(reduction of $FeCl_3$)

Modern Concept of Oxidation and Reduction : According to modern concept, loss of electrons is called oxidation whereas gain of electrons is called reduction. *Example—*

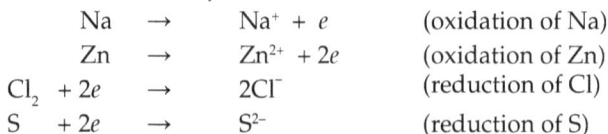

Na	$\rightarrow$	$Na^+ + e$	(oxidation of Na)
Zn	$\rightarrow$	$Zn^{2+} + 2e$	(oxidation of Zn)
$Cl_2 + 2e$	$\rightarrow$	$2Cl^-$	(reduction of Cl)
S $+ 2e$	$\rightarrow$	S^{2-}	(reduction of S)

Oxidising agent (O.A.) : A substance which undergoes reduction is called oxidising agent

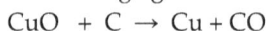

$CuO + C \rightarrow Cu + CO$

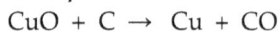

Oxidation – C, Reduction – CuO,   Oxidising agent – CuO

Examples—$O_2, O_3, H_2O_2, KMnO_4, KzCr_2O_7$ etc.

Reducing agent (R.A.) : A substance which undergoes oxidation is called reducing agent.

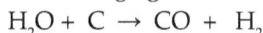

$H_2O + C \rightarrow CO + H_2$

Oxidation — C, Reduction — H_2O,   Reducing agent — C

Examples— $H_2, CO, H_2S, SO_2, C, SnCl_2$ etc.

Redox Reaction : A reaction in which both oxidation and reduction takes place simaltaneously is called redox reaction.

Example—

$CuO + C \rightarrow Cu + CO$

Oxidation – C, Reduction – CuO

Oxidation Number (O.N.) : The charge present on atom in molecule or ion is called oxidation number. It may be zero, positive or negative.

Rules for Determination of Oxidation Number :

(i) Oxidation number of an atom in free state is zero.

(ii) Oxidation number of alkali metals (Li, Na, K, Rb, Cs) in molecule is always + 1.

(iii) Oxidation number of alkaline earth metals (Be, Mg, Ca, Sr, Ba) in a molecule is always + 2

(iv) Oxidation number of hydrogen $\begin{cases} (+1) \text{ hydrogen ion} \\ (-1) \text{ hydride ion} \end{cases}$

(v) Oxidation number of Oxygen $\begin{cases} (-2) \text{ oxide} \\ (-1) \text{ peroxide} \\ -\frac{1}{2} \text{ superoxide} \end{cases}$

(vi) Sum of Oxidation number of atoms in a molecule is equal to zero.

(vii) Sum of oxidation number of atoms in a ion is equal to magnitude of charge with sign.

Oxidation Number of Mn in $KMnO_4$:

Let O.N. of Mn $= x$

$1 + x + (-2) \times 4 = 0$

$$1 + x - 8 = 0$$
$$x = +7$$

Oxidation Number of Cr in $K_2Cr_2O_7$:

Let O.N. of Cr = x

$$1 \times 2 + x \times 2 + (-2) \times 7 = 0$$
$$2 + 2x - 14 = 0$$
$$x = +6$$

Oxidation Number of C in $C_{12}H_{22}O_{11}$:

Let O.N. of C = x

$$x \times 12 + 1 \times 22 + (-2) \times 11 = 0$$
$$12x + 22 - 22 = 0$$
$$x = 0$$

Types of Reactions

1. **Decomposition reactions :** In these reactions, compound either of its own or upon heating decomposes to give two or more components out of which at least one is in the elemental state.

$$2NaH \text{ (s)} \xrightarrow{\Delta} Na \text{ (s)} + H_2 \text{ (g)}$$

$$2H_2O \text{ (1)} \xrightarrow{\Delta} 2H_2 \text{ (g)} + O_2 \text{ (g)}$$

2. **Combination reactions:** In combination reactions, compounds are formed as a result of the chemical combination of two or more elements.

$$H_2 \text{ (g)} + \frac{1}{2}O_2 \text{ (g)} \rightarrow H_2O_2 \text{(l)}$$

$$C \text{ (s)} + O_2 \text{ (g)} \rightarrow CO_2 \text{ (g)}$$
$$3Mg \text{ (s)} + N_2 \text{ (g)} \rightarrow Mg_3N_2 \text{ (s)}$$

3. **Displacement reactions :** In these reactions, an atom/ion present in a compound gets replaced by an atom/ion of another element.

$$FeSO_4 \text{ (aq)} + Zn \text{ (s)} \rightarrow Zn\,SO_4 \text{ (aq)} + Fe \text{ (s)}$$
$$MgO \text{ (aq)} + 2\,Na \text{ (s)} \rightarrow Na_2O \text{ (aq)} + Mg \text{ (s)}$$

4. **Disproportionation reactions :** The chemical reaction in which only one substance is oxidised as well as reduced simultaneously is called disproportionation reaction.

$$Cl_2 + 2NaOH \rightarrow NaCl + NaOCl + H_2O$$
$$P_4 + NaOH + 2H_2O \rightarrow 2NaH_2PO_2 + 2PH_3$$

5. **Substitution reaction :** In these reactions, one or more atoms or groups present in organic molecule get substituted or replaced by suitable atoms or groups.

$$C_2H_2Cl + KOH \text{ (aq)} \rightarrow + C_2H_5OH + KCl$$
Ethyl chloride   Ethyl alcohol

6. **Neutralisation reaction:** When an acid reacts with a base, salt and water is formed. This reaction is called neutralisation reaction.

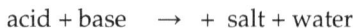

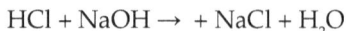

$$acid + base \rightarrow + salt + water$$
$$HCl + NaOH \rightarrow + NaCl + H_2O$$

7. **Reversible reaction :** A reaction in which reactants combine to form products and again products recombine to reactants is called reversible reaction.

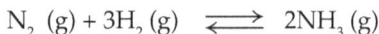

$$N_2\,(g) + 3H_2\,(g) \rightleftharpoons 2NH_3\,(g)$$

8. **Irreversible reaction :** A reaction which proceeds in only one direction is called irreversible reaction.

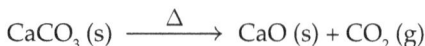

$$CaCO_3\,(s) \xrightarrow{\Delta} CaO\,(s) + CO_2\,(g)$$

6. Acids, Bases & Salts

Acid:

An acid is a substance which

  (i)   is sour in taste
  (ii) tums blue litmus paper into red
  (iii) contains replaceable hydrogen
  (iv) gives hydrogen ion (H^+) in aqueous solution (Arrhenius theorem)
  (v)   can donote a proton (Bronsted & Lowry concept)
  (vi) can accept electron (Lewis theorem)

Uses of acid:

1. As food:
    (a) Citric acid — Lemons or oranges (Citrus fruits}
    (b) Lactic acid — sour milk
    (c) Butyric acid — Rancid butter
    (d) Tarteric acid — Grapes
    (e) Acetic acid — Vinegar
    (f) Maleic acid — Apples
    (g) Carbonic acid — Soda water aerated drinks
    (h) Stearic acid — Fats
    (i) Oxalic and — Tomato, wood sorrel.
2. Hydrochloric acid (HCl) is used in digestion
3. Nitric acid (HNO_3) is used in the purification of gold & silver.
4. Cone. H_2SO_4 and HNO_3 is used to wash iron for its galvanization.
5. Oxalic acid is used to remove rust spot.
6. Boric acid is a constituent of eye wash.
7. Formic acid is present in red ants.
8. Uric acid is present in urine of mammals.

Strength of acids

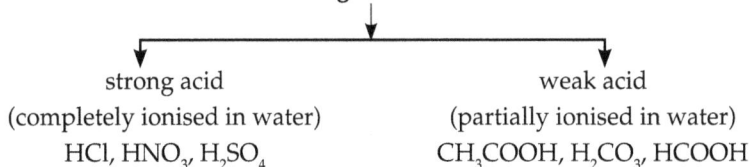

strong acid	weak acid
(completely ionised in water)	(partially ionised in water)
HCl, HNO_3, H_2SO_4	CH_3COOH, H_2CO_3, $HCOOH$

Classification of acids

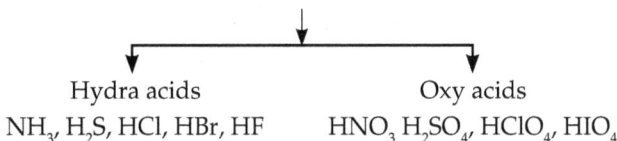

Hydra acids	Oxy acids
NH_3, H_2S, HCl, HBr, HF	HNO_3 H_2SO_4, $HClO_4$, HIO_4

Basicity of an acid : The number of removable hydrogen ions from an acid is called basicity of that acid.

Mono basic acid (one removable H^+ ion) — HCl, HNO_3
Dibasic acid (two removable H^+ ion) — H_2SO_4, H_2CO_3, H_3PO_3
Tribasic acid (three removable H^+ ion) — H_3PO_4
Acidic strength (i) $HF < HCl < HBr < HI$
(ii) $CH_3COOH < H_2SO_4 < HNO_3 < HCl$

Uses of HCl:
(i)   HCl present in gastric juices are responsible for the digestion.
(ii) Used as bathroom cleaner.
(iii) As a pickling agent before galvanization.
(iv) In the tanning of leather.
(v)   In the dying and textile industry.
(vi) In the manufacture of gelatine from bones.

Uses of HNO$_3$
(i)   In the manufacture of fertilizers like ammonium nitrate.
(ii) In the manufacture of explosives like TNT (Trinitro toluene), TNB (Trinitro benzene), Picric acid (Trinitro phenol) etc.
(iii) Nitro glycerine (Dynamite)
(iv) Found in rain water (first shower)
(v)   It forms nitrates in the soil.
(vi) In the manufacture of rayon.
(vii) In the manufacture of dyes & drugs.

Uses of Sulphuric acid (H$_2$SO$_4$)
(i)   In lead storage battery.
(ii) In the manufacture of HCl.
(iii) In the manufacture of Alum.
(iv) In the manufacture of fertilizers, drugs, detergents & explosives.

Use of Boric acids : As an antiseptic.

Uses of Phosphoric acid :

(i)   Its calcium salt makes our bones.

(ii) It forms phosphatic fertilizers.

(iii) PO_4^{-3} is involved in providing energy for chemical reactions in our body.

Uses of Ascorbic acid: Source of Vitamin C

Uses of Citric acid : Flavouring agent & food preservative.

Uses of Acetic acid : Flavouring agent & food preservative.

Uses of Tartaric acid : (i) Souring agent for pickles (ii) A component of baking powder (sodium bicarbonate + tartaric acid)

Indicator properties of an acid

Indicator	Colour changes
Blue litmus paper	turns red
Methyl orange	From orange to pink
Phenolphthalein	Remains colourless

Bases:

A. Base is a substance which:

(i)   bitter in taste

(ii) turns red litmus paper into blue

(iii) gives hydroxyl ions (OH^-) in aqueous solution.

(iv) can accept proton (Bronsted and lowry concept)

(v) can donate electrons (Lewis theory)

➪ Oxides and hydroxides of metals are bases

➪ Water soluble bases are called alkali e.g. NaOH, KOH, etc.

➪ All alkalies are bases but all bases are not alkalies because all bases are not soluble in water.

Indicator properties of an bases

Indicator	Change of colour
Red litmus paper	turns blue
Methyl orange	from orange to yellow
Phenolphthalein	from colourless to pink

Acidity of a base: The number of removable hydroxyl (OH^-) ions from a base is called acidity of a base.

Acidity of NaOH   = 1

Acidity of KOH   = 1

Acidity of $Ca(OH)_2$ = 2

The pH scale : pH of a solution is the negative logarithm of the concentration of hydrogen ions in mole per litre.

$$pH = -\log[H^+]$$

If pH < 7 then solution is acidic

If pH > 7 then solution is basic

The pH value of some common liquids

Liquid	pH
Lemon juice	2.5
Wine	2.8
Apple juice	3.0
Vinegar	3.0
Urine	4.8
Coffee	5.0
Saliva	6.5
Milk	6.5
Blood	7.4
Pure water	7.0
Sea water	8.5
Toothpaste	9.0
Milk of magnesia	10.5

If pH = 7 then solution is neutral

Salt : When an acid reacts with a base, salt and water are formed.

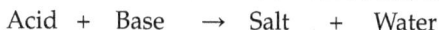

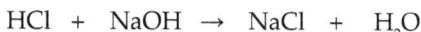

Acid + Base → Salt + Water

$HCl + NaOH \rightarrow NaCl + H_2O$

Uses of some important salts:

1. **Sodium chloride :** As a flavouring agent in food. In saline water for a patient of dehydration (0.9% NaCl), In the manufacture of HCl etc.
2. **Sodium iodate :** Iodised salt to prevent Goitre disease.
3. **Sodium carbonate :** As washing soda, manufacturing of glass etc.
4. **Sodium benzoate :** As a food preservative for pickles.
5. **Potassium nitrate :** As a fertilizer giving both K & N to the solid, In gun powder $(C + S + KNO_3)$, In match sticks etc.
6. **Calcium Chloride :** Dehydrating agent used for removing moisture from gases.
7. **Calcium carbonate (lime stone) :** In the construction of building, In the cement industry. In the extraction of metals etc.
8. **Calcium sulphate :** (i) Plaster of Paris $(2\ CaSO_4 \cdot H_2O)$ – For moulds & statues, in the cement industry in the form of Gypsum $(CaSO_4 \cdot 2H_2O)$.
9. **Calcium phosphate :** As a fertilizer (Superphosphate of lime)
10. **Bleaching powder :** (i) As a disinfectant (ii) As a bleaching agent (removing colours)
11. **Alum (Potassium aluminium sulphate) :** (i) In the purification of water. (ii) In the dyeing industry (iii) As antiseptic after shave.

The acidic and basic nature of some household substances

	Acidic		Basic (Alkaline)
1.	Bathroom acid	1.	Milk of magnesia (Anta acids)
2.	Vitamin C tablets (Ascorbic acid)	2.	Toothpaste
3.	Lemon juice	3.	Soap solution or detergent solution
4.	Orange juice	4.	Solution of washing soda.
5.	Tomato juice	5.	Slaked lime & white wash
6.	Vinegar		
7.	Fizzy drinks (Colas & Sodawater)		

7. Behaviour of Gases

1. **Boyle's law :** At constant temperature, the volume of a definite mass of a gas is inversely proportional to pressure.

    $V \propto \dfrac{1}{p}$ (at constant T) or, $V = K \cdot \dfrac{1}{P}$

    $pV = K$ (where K is a constant)

    $p_1 V_1 = p_2 V_2$

2. **Charle's law :** At constant pressure, the volume of a definite mass of a gas is directly proportional to absolute temperature.

    i.e. $V \propto T$ (at constant p) or, $V = K.T$ or, $\dfrac{V}{T} = k$

    $\therefore \dfrac{V_1}{T_1} = \dfrac{V_2}{T_2}$

3. **Gay-Lussac's law:** At constant volume, the pressure of given mass of a gas is directly proportional to the temp in Kelvin.

    $p \propto T$ (at constant V) or, $p = K.T$

    or, $\dfrac{p}{T} = K$ $\qquad \therefore \dfrac{p_1}{T_1} = \dfrac{p_2}{T_2}$

4. **Avogardds gas law :** At constant temperature and pressure the volume of a gas is directly proportional to the number of molecules.

    $V \propto n$ (at constant T & p)

5. **Ideal gas equation :** $pV = nRT$ is called ideal gas equation. Where

    p = Pressure, $\qquad V$ = volume

    n = number of mole $\quad T$ = temperature in Kelvin

    R = gas constant

    = 0.0821 lit atm K^{-1} mol^{-1}

    = 8.314 J K^{-1} mol^{-1}

    = 1.987 cal K^{-1} mol^{-1}

6. **S.T.P. & N.T.P. :**

    S.T.P. — Standard temperature and pressure.

    N.T.P. — Normal temperature and pressure .

    At S.T.P.; for 1 mole gas

    V = 22.4 litre = 22400 ml

    p = 1 atm = 76 cm of Hg = 760 mm of Hg

    T = 273 K

    Diffusion of gases : The process of intermixing of gases irrespective of the density relationship and without the effect of extemal agency is called diffusion of gases.

In a gas, the molecules are far separated and the empty space among the molecules are very large. Therefore the molecules of one gas can move into the empty spaces or voids of the other gas and vice-versa. This leads to diffusion.

Graham's law of diffusion : Under the similar conditions of temperature and pressure, the rates of diffusion of gases are inversely proportional to the square roots of their densities.

Let r_1 and r_2 be the rates of diffusion of two gases A and B, d_1 and d_2 be their respective densities, then according to Graham's law of diffusion.

$$\frac{r_1}{r_2} = \sqrt{\frac{d_2}{d_1}} = \sqrt{\frac{M_2}{M_1}}$$

Since molecular mass = 2 × vapour density.

$M = 2 \times d$

Dalton's law of partial pressure : It states that — If two or more gases which do not react chemically are enclosed in a vessel, the total pressure of the gaseous mixture is equal to the sum of the partial pressure that each gases which exert pressure when enclosed separately in the same vessel at constant temperature.

Let p_1, p_2 and p_3 be the pressure of three non-reactive gases when enclosed separately. Let total pressure be p

then $\qquad p = p_1 + p_2 + p_3$

8. Electrolysis

1. **Electrolytes :** These are the substances which allow the electricity to pass through them in their molten states or in the form of their aqueous solution and undergo chemical decomposition. *Examples* — acids, bases & salts.

2. **Strong electrolytes :** The electrolytes which are almost completely dissociated into ions in solution are called strong electrolytes. *Example*— NaCl, KCl, HCl, NaOH etc.

3. **Weak electrolytes:** The electrolytes which do not ionise completely in solution are called weak electrolytes. *Example*—CH_3COOH, H_2CO_3, HCN, $ZnCl_2$, NH_4OH etc.

4. **Electrolysis :** The process of chemical decomposition of an electrolyte by passage of electric current through its molten state or its solution is called electrolysis.

5. **Electrodes :** In order to pass the current through an electrolytes in molten state or in aqueous solution, two rods or plates are needed to connect with the terminal of a battery. These rods or plates are called electrodes.

Anode : The electrode which is attached to positive terminal of battery is called anode. Oxidation occurs at anode.

Cathode : The electrode which is attached to negative terminal of batteries is called, Reduction occurs at cathode.

Examples — Electrolysis of molten NaCl

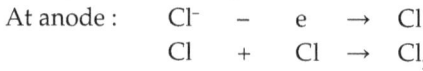

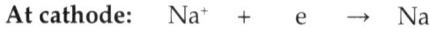

At anode : $\quad Cl^- \quad - \quad e \quad \rightarrow \quad Cl$

$\qquad\qquad\quad Cl \quad + \quad Cl \quad \rightarrow \quad Cl_2$

At cathode: $\quad Na^+ \quad + \quad e \quad \rightarrow \quad Na$

So, Cl_2 gas occurs at anode while Na at cathode.

9. Fuels

A substance that can supply energy either alone or by reacting with another substance is known as fuel. Heat produced by fuel is measured in Calories. An ideal fuel should

(i)   have high calorific value

(ii) be cheap and easily available

(iii) be easily stored & transport

(iv) be regulated and controlled

(v)   have low ignition temperature

The quantity of fuel is expressed in the form of calorific value.

Calorific   value is the total quantity of heat liberated by complete combustion of a unit mass of fuel in air or oxygen.

Calorific value of fuels are expressed in kcal/ m^3 or British Thermal unit (B.T.U) per cubic foot.

$1 \text{ kcal}/m^3 = 0.107 \text{ B.T.U }/ft^3$

Fuel may be sold (e.g wood, coal etc.)

Liquid (e.g kerosene oil, petroleum, alcohol etc.) or gas (e.g water gas, producer gas, coal gas, oil gas, natural gas, gobar gas, LPG etc.) However, gaseous fuel are considered to be the best fuels.

1. Water gas (syn gas) : It is a mixture of carbon monoxide and hydrogen. It is obtained by the action of steam on a red hot coke at 1000°C.

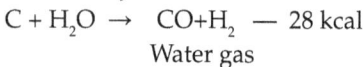

$C + H_2O \quad \rightarrow \quad CO + H_2 \quad - \quad 28 \text{ kcal}$

$\qquad\qquad\qquad$ Water gas

It has a high calorific value (2700 kcal/m^3)

Producer gas : It is a mixture of CO and N_2. It is prepared by burning coke in limited supply of air. It is the cheapest gaseous fuel, however its calorific value is not very high because it has a large proportion of nitrogen.

Coal gas : It is a mixture of H_2, CH_4, CO and other gases like N_2, C_2H_4, O_2 etc. It is obtained by destructive distillation of coal at about 1000°C.

Oil gas : It is a mixture of H_2, CH_4, C_2H_4, CO and other gases like CO_2. It is obtained by thermal cracking of kerosene oil. It is used in laboratories.

Gobar gas : It contains CH_4, CO and H_2. It is produced by fermentation of gobar in absence of air. It is used as a domestic fuel in villages.

Natural gas : It is a mixture of gaseous hydrocarbons viz methane 85%, ethane, propane butane etc. Liquefied petroleum mainly butane and isobutane.

Coal : On the basis of carbon % and calorific value there are four types of coal.

S.N.	Nature	% of carbon	Calorific value
1.	**Peat** : Low grade coal produces less heat & more smoke & ash.	50–60%	2500–3500
2.	**Lignite** : High moisture content burns easily, low calorific value.	60–70%	3500–4500
3.	**Bituminous** : Black, hard, smoky, flame, domestic fuel.	75–80%	7500–8000
4.	**Anthracite** : Superior quality, hardest form, high calorific value.	90–95%	6700–7500

10. Metallurgy

The process of extracting metal in pure form from its ore is known as metallurgy.

Minerals : The compound of a metal found in nature is called a mineral. A mineral may be a single compound or a complex mixture.

Ores : Those minerals from which metal can be economically and easily extracted are called ores.

All ores are mineral but all minerals are not ores.

Gangue (or matrix) : The ore is generally associated with earthy impurities like sand, rocks and limestone known as gangue or matrix.

Flux : A substance added to ore to remove impurities is called flux. There are two types of flux- (i) acidic flux. (ii) basic flux.

Acidic flux is added to remove basic impurity

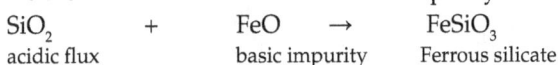

$$\underset{\text{acidic flux}}{SiO_2} + \underset{\text{basic impurity}}{FeO} \rightarrow \underset{\text{Ferrous silicate}}{FeSiO_3}$$

Basic flux is added to remove acidic impurity.

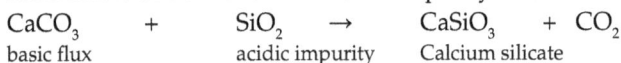

$$\underset{\text{basic flux}}{CaCO_3} + \underset{\text{acidic impurity}}{SiO_2} \rightarrow \underset{\text{Calcium silicate}}{CaSiO_3} + CO_2$$

Slag : Combination of gangue with flux in ores forms a fusible material which is called slag.

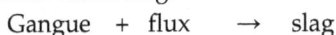

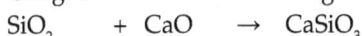

Gangue + flux $\rightarrow$ slag

SiO_2 + CaO $\rightarrow$ $CaSiO_3$

Concentration : The process of removal of gangue from the ore is known as concentration of ore. Concentration of ore can be carried out in the following ways depending upon the nature of the ore.

(i) Gravity separation (ii) Magnetic concentration

(ii) Froth flotation process (iv) Chemical methods

Calcination : Calcination is a process in which ore is heated, generally in the absence of air, to expel water from hydrated oxide or carbon dioxide from a carbonate at temperature below their melting point

Example :

$$Al_2O_3 . 2H_2O \xrightarrow{\Delta} Al_2O_3 + 2H_2O$$

$$CaCO_3 \xrightarrow{\Delta} CaO + CO_2$$

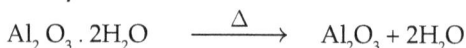

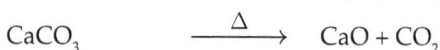

Roasting : Roasting is a process in which ore is heated usually in the presence of air, at temperatures below its melting points.

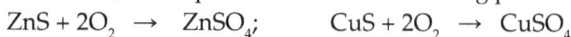

$$ZnS + 2O_2 \rightarrow ZnSO_4; \qquad CuS + 2O_2 \rightarrow CuSO_4$$

Smelting : The reduction of oxide ore with carbon at high temperature is known as smelting.

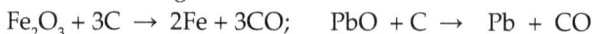

$$Fe_2O_3 + 3C \rightarrow 2Fe + 3CO; \qquad PbO + C \rightarrow Pb + CO$$

Important metals and their ores

Metal	Ores	Chemical Formula
Sodium (Na)	Chile saltpeter	$NaNO_3$
	Trona	$Na_2CO_3, 2NaHCO_3 . 3H_2O$
	Borax	$Na_2B_4O_7 . 10H_2O$
	Common salt	$NaCI$
Aluminium (AI)	Bauxite	$Al_2O_3 . 2H_2O$
	Corundum	Al_2O_3
	Felspar	$K\,AI\,Si_3O_8$
	Cryolite	Na_3AIF_6
	Alunite	$K_2SO_4 . Al_2(SO_4)_3 . 4Al(OH)_3$
	Kaolin	$3AI_2O_3 . 6SiO_2 . 2H_2O$
Potassium (K)	Nitre (salt peter)	KNO_3
	Carnalite	$KCI . MgCl_2 . 6H_2O$
Magnesium (Mg)	Magnesite	$MgCO_3$
	Dolomite	$MgCO_3 . CaCO_3$
	Epsom salt	$MgSO_4 . 7H_2O$
	Kieserite	$MgSO_4 . H_2O$
	Camalite	$KCI . MgCl_2 . 6H_2O$
Calcium (Ca)	Dolomite	$CaCO_3 . MgCO_3$
	Calcite	$CaCO_3$
	Gypsum	$CaSO_4 . 2H_2O$
	Fluorspar	CaF_2
	Asbestus	$CaSiO_3 . MgSiO_3$
Strontium (Sr)	Strontianite	$SrCO_3$
	Silestine	$SrSO_4$

Copper (Cu)	Cuprite	Cu_2O
	Copper glance	Cu_2S
	Copper pyrites	$CuFeS_2$
Silver (Ag)	Ruby Silver	$3\,Ag_2S \cdot Sb_2S_3$
	Horn Silver	$AgCl$
Gold(Au)	Calaverite	$AuTe_2$
	Silvenites	$[(Ag, Au)\,Te_2]$
Barium (Ba)	Barytes	$BaSO_4$
Zinc (Zn)	Zinc blende	ZnS
	Zincite	ZnO
	Calamine	$ZnCO_3$
Mercury (Hg)	Cinnabar	HgS
Tin (Sn)	Casseterite	SnO_2
Lead (Pb)	Galena	PbS
Antimony (Sb)	Stibenite	Sb_2S_3
Cadmium (Cd)	Greenocite	CdS
Bismuth (Bi)	Bismuthite	Bi_2S_3
Iron (Fe)	Haemetite	Fe_2O_3
	Lemonite	$2Fe_2O_3 \cdot 3H_2O$
	Magnetite	Fe_3O_4
	Siderite	$FeCO_3$
	Iron Pyrite	FeS_2
	Copper Pyrites	$CuFeS_2$
Cobalt(Co)	Smelite	$CoAsS_2$
Nickel (Ni)	Milarite	NiS
Magnese (Mn)	Pyrolusite	MnO_2
	Magnite	$Mn_2O_3 \cdot 2H_2O$
Uranium (U)	Carnetite	$K(UO)_2 \cdot VO_4 \cdot 3H_2O$
	Pitch blende	U_3O_8

Alloys : An alloy is a metallic intimately mixed solid mixture of two or more different elements, at least one of which is metal.

Alloys are homogeneous in molten state but they may be homogeneous or heterogeneous in solid state.

Important alloys & their uses

Alloys	Compositions	Uses
Brass	Cu (70%) + Zn (30%)	In making utensils
Bronze	Cu (90%) + Sn (10%)	In making coins, bell and utensils
German Silver	Cu + Zn + Ni (60% + 20% + 20%)	In making utensils
Rolled gold	Cu (90%) + Al (10%)	In making cheap ornaments
Gun metal	Cu + Sn + Zn + Ph (88% 10% 1% 1%)	In making gun, barrels, gears & bearings
Delta metal	Cu + Zn +Fe (60% 38% 2%)	In making blades of aeroplane
Munz metal	Cu (60%) + Zn (40%)	In making coins
Dutch metal	Cu (80%) + Zn (20%)	In making artificial ornaments
Monel metal	Cu (70%) + Ni (30%)	For base containing container
Rose metal	Bi + Pb + Sn (50% 28% 22%)	For making automatic fuse
Solder	Pb (50%) + Sn (50%)	For soldering
Magnalium	AI (95%) + Mg (5%)	For frame of Aeroplane
Duralumin	AI + Cu + Mg + Mn (94% 3% 2% 1%)	For making utensils
Type metal	Sn + Ph + Sb (5% 80% 15%)	In printing industry
Bell metal	Cu (80%) + Sn (20%)	For casting bells, statues
Stainless steel	Fe + Cr + Ni + C (75%, 15%, 10%, 0.05%)	For making utensils and surgical cutlery
Nickel steel	Fe (95%) + Ni (5%)	For making electrical wire, automobile parts

Amalgum : An alloy in which one of the component metals is mercury, is called amalgam.

In alloys, the chemical properties of the component elements are retained but certain physical properties are improved.

Compounds of metal and non-metal and their uses :

1. **Ferrous oxide (FeO) :** In green glass, ferrous salt.
2. **Ferric oxide (Fe_3O_4) :** In electroplating of ornaments and formation of ferric slat.
3. **Ferrous sulphate ($FeSO_4 \cdot 7H_2O$) :** In dye industry, and Mohr's salt.

4. **Ferric hydroxide [(Fe(OH)$_3$)]** : In laboratory reagent and in making medicines.
5. **Iodine (I$_2$)** : (i) As antiseptic, (ii) In making tincture of iodine.
6. **Bromine (Br$_2$)** : (i) In dye industry (ii) As laboratory reagent
7   **Chlorine (Cl$_2$)** : In the formation of (i) Mustard gas (ii) Bleaching powder
8. **Hydrochloric acid (HCl)** : In the formation of aquaregia (3HCl: 1HNO$_3$) and dyes
9. **Sulphuric acid (H$_2$SO$_4$)** : (i) As a reagent (ii) In purification of petroleum (iii) In lead storage battery.
10. **Sulphur dioxide (SO)** : (i) As oxidants and reductants (ii) As bleaching agent
11. **Hydrogen Sulphides (H$_2$S)** : In qualitative analysis of basic radical (group separation)
12. **Sulphur (S)** : Antiseptics, vulcanization of rubber, gun powder, medicine.
13. **Ammonia (NH$_3$)** : As reagent in ice factory.
14. **Phosphorous** : (i) Red (P$_4$) refrigerant, in match industry etc. (ii) White (P$_4$) – Rat killing Medicine.
15. **Producer gas (CO+ N$_2$)** : (i) In heating furnace (ii) Cheap fuel (iii) In Extraction of metal
16. **Water gas (CO+ H)** : (i) As fuel (ii) Welding work
17. **Coal gas** : (i) As fuel (ii) Inert atmosphere
18. **Nitrous oxide (N$_2$O)** : Laughing gas, Surgery.
19. **Carbondioxide (CO$_2$)** : Sodawater, Fire extinguisher.
20. **Carbon monoxide (CO)** : In phosgene gas (COCl$_2$).
21. **Graphite** : As electrodes.
22. **Diamond** : Ornaments, Glass cutting, Rock drilling.
23. **Alum [K$_2$SO$_4$ Al$_2$ (SO4)$_3$·24 H$_2$O]** : (i) Purification of water (ii) Leather industry.
24. **Aluminium sulphate [Al$_2$SO$_4$)$_3$ · 18H$_2$O]** : In paper industry/fire extinguisher.
25. **Anhydrous aluminium chloride (AlCl$_3$)** : Cracking of petroleum.
26. **Mercuric Chloride (HgCl$_2$)** : Calomel, Insecticides (Corrosive sublimate)
27. **Mercuric oxide (HgO)** : Oientment, poison.
28. **Mercury (Hg)** : Thermometer vermillion, amalgam.
29. **Zinc Sulphide (ZnS)** : White pigment.
30. **Zinc Sulphate** (White vitriol) **(ZnSO$_4$ · 7H$_2$O)** Lithopone, Eye ointment.
31. **Zinc Chloride (ZnCl$_2$)** : Textile industry.
32. **Zinc oxide (ZnO)** : Ointment.
33. **Zinc (Zn)** : In battery.
34. **Calcium carbide CaC$_2$)** : Calcium cyanide & acetylene gas.
35. **Bleaching powder [Ca(OCl) Cl]** : Insecticides, Bleaching actions.

36. **Plaster of paris [(CaSO$_4$)$_2$ · 2H$_2$O/CaSO$_4$ ½H$_2$O)]** : Statue, Surgery.
37. **Calcium sulphate (CaSO$_4$ · 2H$_2$O)** : Cement industry.
38. **Calcium carbonate (CaCO$_3$)** : Lime & toothpaste.
39. **Copper sulphate (CuSO$_4$ · 5H$_2$O)** : Insecticides, Electric cells.
40. **Cupric oxide (CuO)** : Blue & green glass, purification of petroleum
41. **Cuprous Oxide (Cu$_2$O)** : Red glass, pesticides.
42. **Copper (Cu)** : Electrical wire.
43. **Sodium nitrate (NaNO$_3$)** : Fertilizer.
44. **Sodium Sulphate (Glauber salt) (Na$_2$SO$_4$·10H$_2$O)** : Medicine, cheap glass
45. **Sodium bicarbonate (Baking soda) (NaHCO$_3$)** : Fire extinguisher, bakery, reagent.
46. **Sodium Carbonate (Washing soda)** : (i) Glass industry (ii) Paper industry (iii) Removal of permanent hardness of water (iv) washing
47. **Hydrogen peroxide (H$_2$O$_2$)** : Oxidants & reductants, Insecticides.
48. **Heavy water (D$_2$O)** : Nuclear reactor.
49. **Liquid hydrogen** : Rocket fuel.

11. Important Facts About Some Metals

➪ Zinc phosphide is used for killing rats.
➪ Wood furnitures are coated with zinc chloride to prevent termites .
➪ Excess of copper in human beings causes disease called Wilson.
➪ Galvanised iron is coated with zinc.
➪ Rusting of iron is a chemical change which increases the weight of iron.
➪ Calcium hydride is called hydrolith.
➪ Calcium hydride is used to prepare fire proof and waterproof clothes.
➪ In flash-blub, magnesium wire is kept in atmosphere of nitrogen gas.
➪ Titanium is called strategic metal because it is lighter than iron.
➪ Group 1st element are called alkali metals because its hydroxides are alkaline whereas group 2nd elements are called alkaline earth metals.
➪ Babbitt metal contains 89% Sn (Tin), 9% Sb (Antimony) and 2% Cu (Copper).
➪ Gun powder contains 75% Potassium nitrate, 10% sulphur and 15% charcoal.
➪ Chromium trioxide is known as chromic acid.
➪ Nichrome wire is used in electrical heater [(Ni, Cr, Fe)]
➪ Potassium carbonate (K$_2$CO$_3$) is known as pearl ash.
➪ Generally transition metals and their compounds are coloured.
➪ Zeolite is used to remove hardness of water.
➪ In cytochrome iron (Fe) is present.
➪ Selenium metal is used in photo electric cell.
➪ Galium metal is liquid at room temperature.
➪ Palladium metal is used in aeroplane.
➪ Radium is extracted from pitchblende.

⇨ World famous Eiffel Tower has steel and cement base.
⇨ Actinides are radioactive elements.
⇨ Cadmium rod is used in nuclear reactor to slow down the speed of neutron.
⇨ Sodium peroxide is used in submarine and also to purify closed air in hospital.
⇨ Co (60) is used in cancer treatment.
⇨ Onion and garlic odour due to potassium.
⇨ Oxides of metals are alkaline.
⇨ Silver and copper are the best conductor of electricity.
⇨ Gold and Silver are the most malleable metal.
⇨ Mercury and iron produces more resistance in comparison to the other during the flow of electricity.
⇨ Lithium is the lightest and the most reductant element.
⇨ In fireworks, crimson red colour is due to presence of strontium (Sr).
⇨ Green colour is due to the presence of Barium in fireworks.
⇨ Barium sulphate is used in X-ray of abdomen as barium meal.
⇨ Barium hydroxide is known as Baryta water.
⇨ Osmium is the heaviest metal and the Platinum is the hardest.
⇨ Zinc oxide is known as flower of zinc. It is also known as chinese white and used as white paint.
⇨ Silver chloride is used in photochromatic glass.
⇨ Silver iodide is used in artificial rain.
⇨ Silver nitrate is used as marker during election. It is kept in coloured bottle to avoid decomposition.
⇨ Silver spoon is not used in egg food because it forms black silver sulphide.
⇨ To harden the gold, copper is mixed. Pure gold is 24 carrat.
⇨ Iron Pyrites (FeS_2) is known as fool's gold.
⇨ Mercury is kept in iron pot because it doesn't form amalgum with iron.
⇨ In tubelight there is the vapour of mercury and argon.
⇨ Tetra-Ethyl lead is used as anti-knocking compound.
⇨ Lead-pipe is not used for drinking water because it forms poisonous lead hydroxide.
⇨ Fuse wire is made up of lead and tin.

12. Non-metal

In modern periodic table there are 24 non metals, 11 are gases, 1 is liquid (Br_2) and 12 are solid.

Electronegative elements are non metals.

Non metals are bad conductor of heat and electricity except graphite, Si & Ge are semi conductor.

Hydrogen (H_2)

The lightest gas having three isotopes

$_1H^1$,	$_1H^2$,	$_1H^3$
Protium	Deuterium	Tritium (Radioactive)

Protium is only one isotope in Periodic Table having zero neutron.

Deuterium oxide is known as heavy water and used in nuclear reactor as moderator.

Liquid hydrogen is used as rocket fuel.

Hydrogen is known as range element because it may kept in group I & group VII A.

Water (H_2O)

Hard water – Less froth with soap

Soft water – more froth with soap.

Hard water – Due to the presence of soluble impurities of bicarbonates, chlorides & sulphates of Ca and Mg.

Temporary hardness – Due to the presence of bicarbonate of calcium and magnesium.

Permanent hardness – Due to the presence of chlorides and sulphates of calcium and magnesium.

Temporary hardness is removed by boiling and by Clark's method while permanent hardness is removed by Soda ash (Na_2CO_3) process.

Permanent hardness is also removed by permutit process.

Oxygen

Important constituent of air, exists in three different isotopes.

$$_8O^{16}, {}_8O^{17}, {}_8O^{18}$$

Ozone (O_3) is the allotrope of Oxygen.

Ozone reduces the effect of ultraviolet rays in the atmosphere.

Nitrogen

78% by volume in atmosphere, liquid nitrogen is used for refrigeration.

Ammonia is an important compound of N_2 which is prepared by Haber's process.

Ammonia

As refrigerent, In the manufacture of HNO_3.

In fertilizer like urea, ammonium sulphate etc.

In the manufacture of Na_2CO_3 & $NaHCO_3$.

In preparation of ammonium salt.

In preparation of explosive.

In prepqration of Artificial silk.

Nitrogen fixation in leguminous plants

Phosphorous

An important constituent of animals and plants. It is present in bones and DNA.

Phosphorous shows allotropy – White or yellow phosphorous, Red phosphorous, Black phosphorous etc.

White phosphorous is more reactive than red phosphorous.

Halogens

17th group elements

Uses of fluorine : In the preparation of UF_6 and SF_6 for energy production and as dielectric constant respectively.

By using HF, chloro fluoro carbon compound and polytetra fluoro ethylene can be synthesised.

Chlorofluoro carbon is known as Freon used as refrigerent and aerosol.

Non-stick utensil is made up of teflon.

Chlorine is used to prepare PVC, insecticides herbicides etc.

Bromine is used in ethylene bromide synthesis which is mixed with leaded pertrol. In the preparation of AgBr which is used in photography.

Inert gases

It belongs to 18th group of P.T.

He, Ne, Ar, Kr, Xe, Rn

Except Rn, all inert gases are present in atmosphere.

Argon is used in Arc. welding & electric bulb.

Helium is light & non-inflammable so, used in balloon, weather indicator etc.

Neon is used in discharge tube glow light.

13. Common Facts

	Catalyst	Process
1.	Fe + Mo	Synthesis of NH_3 by Haber's process.
2.	Ni	Synthesis of vanaspati ghee (hydrogenation)
3.	Pt	Synthesis of H_2SO_4 by Contact process.
4.	NO	In the manufacture of H_2SO_4 by the Lead chamber process.
5.	Hot Al_2O_3	In the preparation of Ether from Alcohol.
6.	$CuCl_2$	Preparation of chlorine gas by Deacon process.

Some Important Explosive

⇨ **Dynamite:** It was discovered Alfred Nobel in 1863. It is prepared by absorption of raw dust with nitro-glycerine. In modern dynamite Sodium Nitrate is used in place of nitro-glycerine.

⇨ Tri Nitro Toluene (TNT)

⇨ Tri Nitro Benzene (TNB)

⇨ Tri Nitro Phenol (TNP) : It is also known as picric acid.

- R.D.X is highly explosive known as plastisizer in which Aluminium powder is mixed to increase the temperature and the speed of fire.

Some Important Facts

- Age of fossils and archeological excavation is determined by radioactive carbon (C^{14}).
- Diamond has maximum refractive index and due to total internal reflection. It has lustre.
- Chloroform in sunlight forms poisonous gas 'Phosgene' ($COCl_2$).
- To decrease the basicity of soil gypsum is used.
- In the preparation of Talcom powder theo phestal mineral is used.
- Potassium chloride is most suitable for the removal of permanent hardness of water.
- To avoid melting of ice gelatine is used.
- When dry ice is heated it is directly converted into gas.
- Saccharine is prepared from toluene.
- Cream is a type of milk in which amount of fat is increased while amount of water decrease.
- From one kilogram of honeybee 3500 calorie energy is produces.
- N_2O is known as laughing gas.
- Bones contain about 58% calcium phosphate.
- Phosphine gas is used in voyage as Holmes signal.
- Chlorine gas bleaches the colour of flower.
- Red phosphorus is used in match industry.
- Urea contains 46% nitrogen.
- In the electroplating of vessel NH_4Cl is used.
- Power alcohol is prepared from mixing pure alcohol in benzene which is used as rocket fuel.
- Artificial perfumes are prepared from Ethyl acetate.
- Urea was the first organic compound synthesised in Laboratory.
- Vinegar contains 10% acetic acid.
- Acetylene is used for light production.
- Ferric chloride is used to stop bleeding.
- Barium is responsible for green colour in fireworks.
- Cesium is used in solar cells.
- Yellow phosphorus is kept in water.
- Sea weeds contains iodine.
- During cooking maximum vitamin is lost.
- For the preparation of silver mirror, glucose is used.
- When cream is separated from milk, it's density increases.
- For artificial respiration mixture of oxygen and helium gas cylinder is used.
- In cold places, to decrease the freezing point ethylene glycol is used.
- Hydrogen peroxide is used for oil paintings .
- Sodium is kept in kerosene oil.
- The heaviest element is Osmium (Os).

- The lightest element, least dense and most reductant is lithium (Li).
- Flourine is the most oxidising agent.
- Silver is the best conductor of electricity.
- Radon is the heaviest gas.
- Polonium has the maximum number of isotopes.
- Sulphuric acid is known as oil of vitriol.
- Noble metals — Ag, Au, Pt, Ir, Hg, Pd, Rh, Ru, and Os.

14. Man made substances

1. **Fertilizers:** The substances added to the soil to make up the deficiency of essential elements are known as fertilizers, these are either natural or synthetic (chemical). For a chemical fertilizer, the following requirements should be met :
   (i) It must be sufficiently soluble in water
   (ii) It should be stable so that the element in it may be available for a longer time.
   (iii) It should contain nothing injurious to plants.

Among the chemical fertilizers the two important categories are :
Phosphatic Fertilizers : All naturally occurring phosphates are orthophosphates, the most abundant of these being rock phosphate $[Ca_3(PO_4)_2]$, which is mostly consumed by the fertilizer industry in the manufacture of 'superphosphate of lime', 'triple superphosphate' and 'nitrophos'— a combined phosphatic and nitrogenous fertilizer. Other phosphatic fertilizers are ammoninum dihydrogen orthophosphate and diammonium hydrogen orthophosphate, which also counteract nitrogen dificiency.

Nitrogenous Fertilizers : Plants need nitrogen for rapid growth and increase in their protein content. For this reason, nitrogenous fertilizers become more important. The chief nitrogeneous fertilizers are ammonium sulphate, calcium cyanamide, sodium nitrate, ammonium nitrate, urea, diammonium phosphate and ammonium phosphate.

2. **Dyes :** Coloured substances used for colouring textiles, foodstuffs, silk, wool, etc. are called dyes.
   Different classes of dyes are given below.
   (i) **Nitro dyes :** These are polynitro derivatives of phenol where nitro group acts as a chromophore and hydroxyl group as auxochrome. These are less important industrially because the colours are not fast.
   (ii) **Azo dyes :** These are an important class of dyes and are characterised by the presence of azo group (— N = N—) as the chromophore. The groups like NH_2, NR_2 or — OH, etc., present in the molecule containing one or more azo groups act as the auxochromes.
   (iii) **Triphenylmethane dyes:** These dyes contain the paraquinoid moiety as a chromophore and —OH, —NH_2 or —NR_2 as auxochrome . These dyes are not fast to light and washing and hence are mainly used for

colouring paper or typewriter ribbons, e.g. malachite green which is used for dyeing Wool and silk directly and cotton after mordanting with tannin.

(iv) Mordant dyes : Those dyes which are fixed on the fibre with the help of a mordant are known as mordant dyes. For acidic dyes, basic mordants such as hydroxides of iron, aluminium and chromium) are used, while for basic dyes, acidic mordants (like tannic acid) are used. Here the fabric is first dipped into a solution of mordant and then into the dye solution. The colour produced depends on the nature of the mordant used.

(v) Vat dyes : These are water insoluble dyes and are introduced into the fibre in its (soluble) reduced form, also known as *leuco* form (colourless). These are called vat dyes because reducing operation (using sodium hydrosulphite) was formerly carried out in wooden vats. Indigo is a vat dye and is used for dyeing cotton.

Cement: It is a complex material containing the silicates of calcium and aluminium. A paste of it in water sets into a hard rocky mass-called the setting of cement. A paste of sand, cement and water called mortar, is very conveniently used for joining bricks and plastering walls.

A mixture of stone chips (gravel) sand cement and water, known as concrete. Sets harder than ordinary mortar. It is used for flooring and making roads. Concrete with steel bars and wires called reinforced concrete (RC) forms a very strong material. It is used for constructing roofs, bridges and pillars.

Glass : Supercooled liquid is called glass. SiO_2 is it's common constituent.

(a) Soda glass or soda lime glass : It is Sodium calcium silicate (Na_2O CaO 5SiO_2). It is the cheapest of all glasses and used for making window panes and bottles and easily attacked by chemicals.

(b) Potash glass : It contains potassium in place of sodium. it has higher softening temperature as also a greater resistance to chemicals. So used for chemical apparatus; beakers, flasks, funnels etc.

(c) Optical glass : It is used for making lenses, prisms and optical instruments like telescopes and microscopes. It contains boric oxide (B_2O_3) and silica (SiO_2)

Types : **(i) Crown glass :** Contains K_2O & BaO as the basic oxide

(ii) Flint glass : Contains PbO as the basic oxide.

(d) Crooks glass: for spectacles : Absorbs ultraviolet rays which are harmful for the eyes.

(e) Lead crystal and crystal glass : Lead glass sparkles used for making decorative items. It contains 24% or more of PbO called lead crystal. If it contains term than 24% lead oxide called crystal glass.

(f) Borosilicate glass : It contains less alkali (K_2O or CaO_3) and more SiO_2 than potash glass and some B_2O.

(g) Coloured glass :

Colour	Substance added to the glass melt
Red	Selenium (Se) or copper (I) oxide (Cu_2O)
Green	Chromium III oxide (Cr_2O_3)
Violed	Maganese IV oxide (MnO_2)
Blue	Copper II oxide eno or cobalt II oxide (CoO)
Brown	Er on III oxide (Fe_2O_3)

It is used for making artificial jewellery, crockery and stained glass windows.

(h) Milky glass : Milky glass is prepared by adding tin oxide (SnO_2). Calcium phosphate ($Ca_3(PO_4)_2$) or cryolite (AH_33NaF) to the melt glass. All these substances are white so look milky.

(i) Glass laminates : It is made by fixing polymer sheets between layers of glass. It is used to make windows & Screens of cars, trains and aircraft specially manufactured glass laminates are used bulletproof material.

Some common man-made polymers and their uses

Polymer	Use
Polythene	Packaging material, carry bags, bottles.
Polypropene	Bottles, crates
Polyvinyl chloride (PVC)	Pipes insulation
Nylon (Polyester)	Fibres, ropes
Teflon	Nonstick kitchen ware
Vinyl rubber	Rubber erasers
Polystyrene	Foam thermocole
Poly (Styrene butadiene)	Rubber bubble gum
Bakelite	Electrical insulation buttons
Lexan	Bulletproof glass
Melamine	Crockery

Paints : Chemical, contains a pigment as a vehicle and a thinner.

White pigment : Zinc oxide, white lead and titanium dioxide. The pigment is mixed with a vehicle, which is an oil like *linseed* or *soya bean oil* or a *polymer*. A thinner is a solvent such as *turpentine oil* or *kerosene*.

Luminous paints : Glow when exposed to light. Paints are applied on a surface to protect it from corrosion and weathering or to give it an attractive look.

Soaps and Detergents : Soaps are the sodium or potassium salts of fatty acids.They are made by the saponification of fats. Detergents are made from some petroleum products.

Antibiotic : Medicinal compounds produced by moulds and bacteria, capable of destroying or preventing the growth of bacteria in animal systems.

Antibody : Kinds of substances formed in the blood, tending to inhibit or destroy harmful bacteria, etc.

Antidote : Medicine used against a poison, or to prevent a disease from having effect.

Antigen : Substance capable of stimulating formation of antibodies.

Antimony : A brittle, crystalline, silvery white metal.

Antipyretie : A substance used to lower body temperature.

Pesticides : Many living organism destroy crops or eat away grains. They are collectively known as pests. To kill chemical used called pesticides.

Insecticides : D.D.T. aluminium phosphate gammexine.

Fungicide : Thiram, Bordeanx mixture $CaCaSO_4 5H_2O + (OH)_2$

Rodenticides : Aluminium phosphide.

Herbicides : Benzipram, benzadox.

Medicines : To cure diseases by biological changes in the body.

Analgesics : Painkillers are called analgesics eg, Aspirin, Paracetamol and morphine.

Antimalarial drugs : Used to treat malaria quinine derivatives eg, chlorovoquine.

Destroy microorganism : Penicillin, Aminogly considers, oftoxaim, Homophonic.

Sulphadrugs : Alternatives of antibiotics, sulphanilamide, sulphadiazine, Sulpha gunamidine.

Antaoxide : Substances which remove the excess acid and raise the pH to appropriate level in scotch are called *antacids*. It is caused by excess of HCl in the gastric juice magnesium hydrate, magazines carbonate, magnesium truistical, aluminium phosphene are common antacids.

Epsom salt : Hydrated magnesium sulphate ($MgSO_4 \cdot 7H_2O$), used in medicines to empty bowels.

Chloroform : A sweetish, colourless liquid. It is used as a solvent and anaesthetic.

Saccharin : A white crystalline solid which is 550 times sweeter than sugar, but does not have any food value. It is used by diabetic patients.

DDT : Dichloro diphenyl tricholoro ethane, a white powder used as an insecticide.

Biology

1. Introduction

Biology : Branch of science in which living beings are studied.

Bios = Life & Logos = Study. Therefore study of life is called *biology*. The term *biology* was first coined by *Lamarck* and *Treviranus* in the year 1801. Biology has two main branch.

1.   **Botany:** Study of different aspects of plants. *Theophrastusis* known as father of Botany.

2.   **Zoology :** Study of various aspects of animals. *Aristotle* is called father of Zoology as well as Biology.

Important Terms of Biology :

➪ **Anatomy :** Study of internal structure of organism.

➪ **Agrology :** Soil science dealing specially with production of crop.

➪ **Agronomy :** Science of soil management and production of crop.

➪ **Agrostology :** Study of grass.

➪ **Arthrology :** Study of joints.

➪ **Apiculture :** Rearing of honey bee for honey.

➪ **Anthropology :** Study of origin, development and relationship between the culture of past and present human.

➪ **Anthology :** Study of flower and flowering plant .

➪ **Angiology :** Study of blood vascular system including arteries and veins.

➪ **Andrology :** Study of male reproductive organ.

➪ **Bryology :** Study of Bryophytes.

➪ **Biometrics :** Statical study of Biological problem.

➪ **Biomedical engineering :** Production and designing of spare part for overcoming various defects in man. e.g. artificial limbs, Iron lung, Pacemaker etc.

➪ **Biotechnology :** Technology concerned with living beings for wilful manipulation on molecular level.

➪ **Bacteriology :** Study of bacteria.

➪ **Cytology :** Study of cell.

➪ **Cryobiology :** It is the study of effect of low temperature on organisms and their preservation.

➪ **Clone :** Clones are geneticaly identical individual in a population.

➪ **Cardiology :** Study of heart.

➪ **Demography :** Study of population.

➪ **Diffusion :** Random movement of molecule/ion or gases from a region of higher concentration to lower concentration.

➪ **Dermatology :** Study of skin.

➪ **Dendrochronology :** Counting and analysing annual growth rings of tree to know its age.

➪ **Ecology :** Study of inter-relationship between living and their environment.

- ➪ **Evolution** : Study of origin of life, variation and formation of new species.
- ➪ **Embryology** : Study of fertilization of egg, formation of zygote and development of embryo.
- ➪ **Eugenics** : Study of factors connected with the improvement of human race.
- ➪ **Euthenics** : Study of environmental condition that contribute to the improvement of human beings.
- ➪ **Euphenics** : Treatment of defective in heredity through genetics engineering.
- ➪ **Ethnology** : Study of science dealing with different races of human.
- ➪ **Ethology** : Study of animal behaviour in their natured habitats.
- ➪ **Etiology** : Study of causative agent of disease.
- ➪ **Entomology** : Study of insects.
- ➪ **Exobiology** : Study of possibility of life in space.
- ➪ **Floriculture** : Cultivation of plant for flower.
- ➪ **Food technology** : Scientific processing, preservation, storage and transportation of food.
- ➪ **Forensic science** : Application of science for identification of various facts of civilian.
- ➪ **Fishery** : Catching, breeding, rearing and marketing of fishes.
- ➪ **Forestry** : Development and management of forest.
- ➪ **Fermentation** : Process of incomplete oxidation that occur in microbes and other cells in absence of oxygen, leading to the formation of ethyl alcohol.
- ➪ **Genetics** : Study of variation and transmission of heredity character from parents to their young ones.
- ➪ **Growth** : Permanent increase in weight, volume and size of an organism.
- ➪ **Genetic Engineering** : Manipulation of gene in order to improve the organism.
- ➪ **Gynecology** : Study of female reproductive organ.
- ➪ **Gerontology** : Study of ageing.
- ➪ **Gastroenterology** : Study of alimentary canal or stomach, intestine and their disease.
- ➪ **Hypertonic** : When two solutions have higher solute concentration. The solution which have higher concentration is called hypertonic.
- ➪ **Hypotonic** : In two solutions which have lower solute concentration is called hypotonic.
- ➪ **Homeothermic** : Animals who have constant body temperature are called home thermic or warmblooded animal.
- ➪ **Histology** : Study of tissue organisation and their internal structure with the help of microscope.
- ➪ **Hygiene** : Science taking care of health.
- ➪ **Hydroponics** : Study of growing plant without soil in water which contain nutrient.
- ➪ **Haematology** : Study of blood.

- ⇨ **Hepatology :** Study of liver.
- ⇨ **Ichthyology :** Study of fishes.
- ⇨ **Immunology :** Study of immun system or resistance of body to disease.
- ⇨ **Kalology :** Study of human beauty.
- ⇨ **Metazoans :** All multicellular animals are called metazoans.
- ⇨ **Monoecious :** Plant which have both male and female flower
- ⇨ **Morphology :** Study of external structure.
- ⇨ **Microbiology :** Study of micro-organism like virus, bacteria, algae, fungi and protozoa.
- ⇨ **Molecular biology :** Study of molecule found in the body of living organism.
- ⇨ **Medicine :** Study of treating disease by drug.
- ⇨ **Mammography :** Branch of science which deal test of breast cancer.
- ⇨ **Mycology :** Study of fungi.
- ⇨ **Nutrients :** Chemical substance taken as food which are necessary for various function, growth and heath of living.
- ⇨ **Neurology :** Study of nervous system.
- ⇨ **Neonatology :** Study of new born.
- ⇨ **Nephrology :** Study of kidneys.
- ⇨ **Osmosis :** Movement of water molecule across semipermeable membrane from the region of its higher concentration to the region of lower communication.
- ⇨ **Odontology :** Study of teeth and gum.
- ⇨ **Osteology :** Study of bones.
- ⇨ **Oncology :** Study of cancer and tumours.
- ⇨ **Obstetrics :** Science related with care of pregnant women before, during and after child birth.
- ⇨ **Ornithology :** Study of birds.
- ⇨ **Ophthalmology :** Study of eyes.
- ⇨ **Orthopaedics :** Diagnosis and repair of disorder of locomotery system.
- ⇨ **Phytoplanlktons :** Microscopic organism which passively float on the surface of water.
- ⇨ **Parasite :** Organism which depend on other living organism for their food and shelter.
- ⇨ **Poikilothermic :** Organism which change their body temperature according to surrounding. These are also called cold blooded animal.
- ⇨ **Pigment :** A substance which absorb light of certain wavelength like chlorophyll found in green leaves.
- ⇨ **Paleontology :** Study of fossils.
- ⇨ **Physiology :** Study of function of various system of organism.
- ⇨ **Pathology :** Study of diseases, effects, causable agents and transmission of pathogens.
- ⇨ **Pomology :** Study of fruit and fruit yielding plant.
- ⇨ **Psychiatry :** Treatment of mental disease.
- ⇨ **Psychology :** Study of human mind and behavior.
- ⇨ **Pisciculture :** Rearing of fishes.

⇨ **Phycology :** Study of algae.
⇨ **Paediatrics :** Branch of medicine dealing with children.
⇨ **Parasitology :** Study of parasites.
⇨ **Photobiology :** Effect of light on various biological processes.
⇨ **Phylogeny :** Evolutionary history of organism.
⇨ **Physiotherapy :** Treatment of body defects through massage and exercise.
⇨ **Radiology :** Science dealing with the effect of radiation on living beings.
⇨ **Rhinology :** Study of nose and olfactory organs.
⇨ **Sonography :** Study of ultrasound imaging.
⇨ **Saurology :** Study of lizards.
⇨ **Serology :** Study of serum, interaction of antigen and antibodies in the blood.
⇨ **Sphygmology :** Study of pulse and arterial pressure.
⇨ **Taxonomy :** Study of classification, nomenclature and identification of organism.
⇨ **Telepathy :** Communication of thoughts ot ideas from one mind to another without normal use of senses. In other word this is the process of mental contact.
⇨ **Veterinary Science :** Science of health care and treatment of domestic animals.

2. What is Living?

⇨ The word living cannot be defined .
⇨ There are certain characters by which can be distinguished from non living.
   (i) Growth : Increase in the number of cell or mass is called growth
   (ii) Reproduction : Living organism produce young ones of their same kind.
   (iii) metabolism : Chemical reaction occurring inside a living cell.
   (iv) Response of stimuli : Living have the ability to sense the condition of their surrounding and respond to these stimuli.

3. Classification of Organism

⇨ There are millions of organisms. It is impossible to study each individual separately. Classification means to categories organism into different groups. Study of an individual of a group gives us the idea of rest of the member of that group.
⇨ *Linnaeus* divide all organism into two kingdoms – *Planate* and *Animalia* in his book *"System a Nature"*. The foundation of modern classification system was laid in the line of classification system started by *Linnaeus*. Therefore *Linnaeus* is called *'Father of Taxonomy'*. Due to disputed position of organism like bacteria, virus, fungi and euglena, there is need of reconsideration of system of classification.

Five Kingdom Classification

⇨ Five Kingdom Classification was proposed in 1969 by *R.H. Whittaker*. The criteria of classifying organism into five kingdoms are its complexity of *cell structure, complexity of body of organism, mode of nutrition, life style and phylogenetic relationship.*

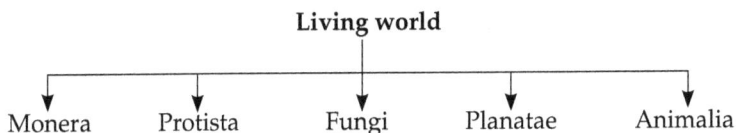

Living world

Monera   Protista   Fungi   Planatae   Animalia

1. **Monera:** It includes all prokaryotic organism like bacteria, cynobacteria and archiobactera. Filamentous bacteria also come under this kingdom. All organism of this kingdom are microscopic.

2. **Protista :** This kingdom includes unicellular form usually found in aquatic habitats. On the basis of mode of nutrition they are autotrophic, parasitic, and saprophytic. Diatoms flagellates and protozoa come under this kingdom. *Euglena* have both heterotrophic and autotrophic mode of nutrition. So, it is placed between plant and animal.

3. **Fungi:** This kingdom includes non-green plants. It has saprophytic nutrition and growing on dead and decaying organic matter. The cell wall is composed of chitin. ***Example*** : *Mushroom, Mucor, Albugo* etc.

4. **Planatae :** This kingdom includes all plants except some algae, diatoms, fungi and member of monera and protista.

5. **Animalia :** Almost all animal comes under this kingdom except protozoan.

⇨ **Binomial nomenclature :** There was the need of uniform international naminging of organism. In biology every organism is given two proper names. The first name is *genus* name always started with capital letter and the second name is *species* started with small letter. For example scientific name of human is *Homo sapiens*. *Homo* is the name genus, whose one *species* is sapiens.

Scientific Names of some Organisms

Man	*Homo sapiens*	Frog	*Rana tigrina*
Cat	*Felis domestica*	Dog	*Canis familaris*
Cow	*Bos indicus*	Housefly	*Musca domestica*
Mango	*Mangifera indica*	Rice	*Oryza sativa*
Wheat	*Triticum aestivum*	Pea	*Pisum sativum*
Gram	*Cicer arietinum*	Mustard	*Brassica campestris*

4. Study of Cell

- **Cell :** Cell is the basic structural and functional unit of life.
- The word 'cell' was first coined by British scientist *Robert Hook* in thi year 1665.
- The smallest cell is *Mycoplasma gallisepticum*.
- The longest cell is *Neuron*.
- The biggest cell is egg of *Ostrich*.
- Schilden and Schwan established cell theory in the year 1838-39.

Main features of the cell theory :

1. All organism are composed of cell.
2. Body of every organism is made of cell.
3. Each cell arises from pre-existing cell.
4. Every organism starts its life from single cell.

Cell is of two kinds

1. **Prokaryotic cell :** These are primitive cell having three basic structure of typical cell but lack nuclear membrane. Nuclear material is present in a region of cytoplasm called *nucleoid*. Other membrane bound organelles are absent such as mitochondria, ribosome, golgi bodies etc. Ex.- Virus, bacteria and cynobacteria are Prokaryotes.
2. **Eukaryotic cell:** These are complete cell which contain membrane bound organelles and nucleus. Unicellular and multicellular plant and animal have Eurkaryotic cell.

Difference between Prokaryotes and Eukaryotes

S.No.	Prokarvotes	S.No.	Eukaryotes
1.	Size of cell is generally large.	1.	Size of cell is generally small.
2.	Nucleus present.	2.	Nucleus absent.
3.	It contain single chromosome which is circular in shape.	3.	It contains more than one chromosome.
4.	Membrane bound cell organelles are absent.	4.	Cell organelles present.
5.	Cell division takes place by fission or budding.	5.	Cell division takes place by mitosis and meiosis.

- **Structure of typical cell:** A cell have following structure.
    1. **Cell wall:** In plant cell there is a rigid cell wall which is non living and freely permeable. It is made up of *cellulose* and *chitin*. It provide shape and rigidity to the cell.
    2. **Cell membrane:** It is also known as *plasma membrane* which form the outer covering of animal cell. In plant cell it is found within cell wall. It is thin, elastic, living, double layer, permeable membrane. It is made up of phospholipid molecules.

Function : It regulates movement of molecules inside and outside of the cell.

3. **Protoplasm** : The whole fluid present inside plasma-membrane is protoplasm. The name protoplasm is given by *Purkenjein* 1839. Protoplasm is made up of various chemical substances like water, ions, salt and organic molecule. It is the living part of cell. Protoplasm is divided into two parts.

   A. **Cytoplasm** : The fluid found outside the nuclear membrane.

   B. **Nucleoplasm** : The fluid found inside the nuclear membrane.

4. **Mitochondria** : Discovered by *Altman* in the year 1886. These are cylindrical, rod shaped or spherical structure found in cytoplasm. It is surrounded by double layered membrane. Inner membrane has many fold called *cristae*. The fluid present inside mitochondria is called *matrix*, which contain many enzyme and co-enzyme.

   Function : Mitochondria is the respiratory site of cellular respiration. Mitochondria synthesize energy rich compound ATP. It is also known as "Power Hosue" of the cell.

5. **Golgi bodies** : Discovered by scientist *Camilo Golgi*. Golgi bodies are made up of group of tubes, vesicles and vacuoles. In plant it is more in number and here it is known as dictyosomes.

   Function : It work as storage, processing and packaging of material. It also involved in the synthesis of cell wall, plasma membrane and lysosomes.

6. **Endoplasmic reticulum** : Membranous network of tubules like structure found in cytoplasm is called *endoplasmic reticulum*. It is attached with the nucleus on one side and on other side it is joined with plasma membrane.

   Function : Endoplasmic reticulum helps in the distribution of material. It forms supporting framework of cell.

7. **Ribosome** : Discovered by *Palade*. Small granules like structure found attached to the endoplasmic reticulum or in free state. It is made up of ribonucleic acid. (RNA)

   Function : Take part in protein synthesis.

8. **Lysosome** : Discovered by *De Duve*. These are sac like structure bounded by single membrane and contain hydrolytic enzyme.

   Function : It helps in intracellular digestion. The enzyme found in tysosome may digest the entire cell. So it is also known as suicidal bag.

9. **Centrosome** : Discovered by *Boveri*. It is only found in animal cell faking part in cell division. It is not bounded by membrane consist of two centriole.

Function : Help in the formation of spindle fibre during cell division.

10. **Plastid** : Only found in plant cell. It is of three type : (a) Chloroplast (b) Chromoplast (c) Leucoplast.

(a) **Chloroplasts** : These are green pigment found in green plant involve in photosynthesis. So, it is known as '*Kitchen of the cell*'. Chloroplast is bounded by two unit membrane having grana and stroma. Grana are membrane bounded sac like structure found in stacks containing chlorophyll molecule. Stroma is the matrix present inside the chloroplast which contain photosynthetic enzymes and starch grain. Granum is the site of light reaction during photosynthesis while stroma is the site of dark reaction.

Function : Chloroplast provides green colour to plant & take part in photosynthesis.

(b) *Chromoplast* provides various colours to the plant.

(c) **Leucoplast** is colourless. It stores the food in the form of starch, fat & protein.

11. **Vacoule** : These are fluid filled single membrane bounded, dead organelles of cell. In plant cell it is larger in size but in animal it is smaller in size.

Function : It helps in osmoregulation. It stores toxic metabolic waste.

12. **Nucleus** : The nucleus is a spherical, centrally located is a major structure found in the cell. In plant cell it is shifted towards periphery. It is bounded by double layered nuclear membrane having pore. Within nucleoplasm nucleolus and chromatin material is present. Nucleolus is rich in protein and RNA. Chromatin material is thin thread like structure forming network. This is made up of genetic substance DNA (deoxyribo nucleic acid) and histone protein. During cell division chromatin breaks into pieces and forms chromosome.

Function: It controls all the activity of cells. So it is also known as "control room "of cell. Chromatin transmits hereditary characters from parents to their offspring.

Difference between Plant and Animal cells Plant cell

Plant cell	Animal Cell
1. Plant cells are larger in size.	1. Animal cells are generally smaller in size.
2. Cell wall present, made up of cellulose and chitin.	2. Cell wall absent

3.	Plastid present.	3.	Plastid absent
4.	Centrosome absent.	4.	Centrosome present
5.	Vacoules are larger in size.	5.	Vacuoles are smaller in size

Chromosome

⇨ Chromosome is thread like structure found in the nucleus. It becomes visible during cell division. Each chromosome is made up of two chromatids joined together at a point centromere. Bead like structure found on chromosome is called *gene*. Genes are made up of DNA (deoxyribo nucleic acid) which is the carrier of genetic information from generation to generation. In some viruses RNA is the genetic material called *rietrovirus*. In prokaryotes there is only one chromosome, like bacteria and viruses.

⇨ Eukaryotic cell posses many chromosome. A particular kind of species have definite number of chromosome in their cell, which are in pair Icnown as *diploid*. The set of unpaired chromosome is called *haploid*. Gametes have haploid set of chromosome.

Number of chromosome in different organism

Pegion	40 pairs	Dog	39 pairs	Horse	32 pairs
Chimpanzee	24 pairs	Human	23 pairs	Wheat	21 pairs
Cat	19 pairs	Frog	13 pairs	Tomato	12 pairs
Onion	8 pairs	Pea	7 pairs	Ascaris	1 pairs

⇨ **Nucleic Acid:** Nucleic acid is complex organic compound found in cell. It contains special genetic instruction in coded form. Nucleic acids are of two kinds.

A. Deoxyribo nucleic Acid (DNA): *Frederic Meischer* was the first who isolated DNA from the nucleus of pus cells. DNA is a macromolecule in which large number of nucleotides are present. Chemically a nucleotide has three components. (1) Nitrogen base (2) Sugar (3) Phosphate group.

⇨ Nitrogen base are of two type—*Purines & Pyrimidines*. Purines contain two nitrogen base—*A dinine and Guanine*. Pyrimidine nitrogen base are *Thymine* and *Cytosine*. Thus there are four kinds of nucleotides present in DNA.

Watson and *Crick* give the structural model of DNA —

1. DNA molecule is consists of two polynucleotide strand, forming a *double helix*. Each strand has a backbone of sugar and phosphate. Nitrogen base is attached to the sugar.

2. Nitrogenous base of the two strands of a double helix form a pair with the help of hydrogen bonds. Adenine pairs with thymine

where as guanine pairs with cytosine. Adenine and thymine are complementary to each other and cytosine is complementary to guanine. Hydrogen bonding between nitrogenous base holds the two strands together. This structure can be compared with the steps of spiral staircase.

Function :   1.   It contains genetic information in coded form.

2.   DNA synthesis RNA.

Note : *DNA is mainly found in nucleus. In small amount it is also found in mitochondria and chloroplast.*

Gene : Gene is hereditary unit which is made by a segment of DNA found on the chromosome.

B. Ribonucleic Acid (RNA): RNA is single stranded nucleic acid made up of phosphate, ribose sugar and nitrogen base uracil, adinine, guanine and cytosine. It is found in nucleus as well as cytoplasm. RNA is of three kind.

1.   **Messenger RNA (*m*RNA):** It brings the massage from DNA found in the nucleus to cytoplasm in the coded form.

2.   **Ribosomal RNA (*r*RNA) :** Present in ribosome which is the site of Protein synthesis.

3.   **Transfer RNA (t RNA):** It is the carrier of amino acid and transfer it to the ribosome.

Function : Synthesis of protein.

Difference between RNA and DNA

DNA	RNA
1. Sugar is deoxyribose type.	1. Sugar is ribose type.
2. It contains the base adenine, thymine and cytosine and guanine.	2. It contains uracil in place of thymine.
3. It is double stranded structure.	3. It is single stranded structure.
4. It is mainly found in nucleus.	4. It is found in both nucleus and cytoplasm.

➪   **Cell cycle:** It is the sequence of events in which cell duplicates its genetic material, synthesis the other constituents of cell and ultimately divide into two daughter cell.

➪   **Cell Division :** The process in which cell increase in their number is cell division. It is needed for growth, development and repair of body. There are mainly two kind of cell division.

A. Mitosis : Mitosis cell division occur in somatic cell which take part in growth, repair and development. In unicellular organism asexual reproduction takes place by this type of cell division.

➪ **Significance of Mitosis :**
1. After Mitosis cell division one cell divided into two daughter cell in which number of chromosome is equal to the parent cell.
2. Uncontrolled Mitosis may cause tumor or cancerous growth.

B. Meiosis : 1. Meiosis cell division occur in reproductive cell. This type of division takes place during the formation of haploid gamete, i.e. ova & sperm.

2. It is also known as *reduction division* during which each daughter cell have haploid number of chromosome.

3. Four daughter cells are produced from one meiotic cell division.

Terms related to cytology :
➪ **Karyokinesis :** Division of nucleus during cell division called Karyok-inesis.
➪ **Cytokinesis :** Division of cytoplasm called *cytokinesis.*
➪ **Diploid :** Two complete set of chromosome is called *diploid*, found in somatic cell.
➪ **Haploid :** Single set of chromosome in cell is called *haploid* found in gametes.
➪ **Crossing over :** Exchange of genetic material between two non sister chromatids takes place during meiosis cell division is called *crossing over.*
➪ **Homologous chromosome :** A pair of chromosome having same size and shape bearing corresponding gene.
➪ **Phenotype :** The character of organism which can be seen directly.
➪ **Genotype :** Genetic constitution of organism is called genotype.
➪ **Tonoplast:** The membrane surrounding the vacuole.
➪ **Unit membrane :** The basic trilamilar structure of cell membrane.

5. Genetics

The process of transfer of hereditry character from one generation to next generation is called *Genetics. Johan Mendel* is known as *father of genetics.* Mendel experiments were based on cross breeding of two pea plant having contrasting characters for same feature i.e. tall and dwarf character of plant are for height of plant. He extended his work by two or three pair of contrasting characters called *dihybrid* and *trihybrid cross.* He concludes some result on the basis of his experiment called *Mendel's law.*

1. **Law of paired unit :** Mendel proposed that when two dissimilar unit factors are present in an individual only one is able to express. One that expresses itself is *dominant unit factor* while other which fails to express is *recessive unit factor.* For example tallness is dominant over dwarfness.

2. **Law of dominance** : Offspring of cross breed parent only show dominant characters in F_1 generation.

3. **Law of segregation** : In F_2 generation both the character which is governed by gene is separated.

4. **Law of independent assortment:** During dihybrid and tribhybrid cross two or three pair of characters are taken. These characters segregate separately without depending on other in F_2 generation.

Term related to genetics :

➪ **Linkage** : Linkage is an exception of Mendel law. When two different gene are present on the same chromosome their effects take place together insted of independently. This phenonmenon is known as *Linkage*. The word linkage first coined by Morgan.

➪ **Mutation** : A sudden change in the gene which is heritable from one generation to other. The term Mutation was first coined by Hugo de *Vries*.

➪ **Variation:** When characters are transmitted from one generation to next generation there is some change. Change in characters by recombination of gene in offspring takes place they looks different from their parents. This phenomenon is known as *Variation*.

➪ **Chromosomal aberrations** : Any change in chromosomal structure is known as *Chromosomal aberrations*.

➪ **Cloning** : It is a process of producing many identical organism from a single cell having same genetic character as his mother. Ex: *Sheep Dolly* was produced from single cell.

➪ **Totipotency** : It is the potential ability of a plant cell to grow into a complete plant.

➪ **Pluriopotency** : It is the potential ability of a cell to develop any kind of the cell of animal body.

➪ **Genetically modified organism (GMO):** Manipulation of gene by cutting or joining the segment of DNA to get desired varieties of organism is called *genetically modified organism*. This is also known as *genetic engineering*.

➪ **Autosomes** : Chromosomes found in cell which are responsible for characters other than sex are called *autosomes*.

➪ **Sex Chromosome** : The pair of chromosome which determine the sex of organism is called *sex-chromosome*.

Human have 23 pair of chromosome in which 22 pair are autosome and 1 pair is sex chromosome.

➪ **Genome** : All gene present in a haploid cell is called *genome*.

6. Sex Determination in Human

➪ In human male sex chromosome is 'XY', where as in female sex chromosome is XX. During gamete formation in male half of the sperm contain 'X' chromosome while other half contain 'Y' Chromosome. In female all gametes contain only one type of chromosome that is 'X'. Thus when a male gamete i.e. sperm carrying 'X' chromosome fertilize an ova, the zygote develop into female. When a sperm carrying 'Y' chromosome fertilizes an egg, zygote develops into male.

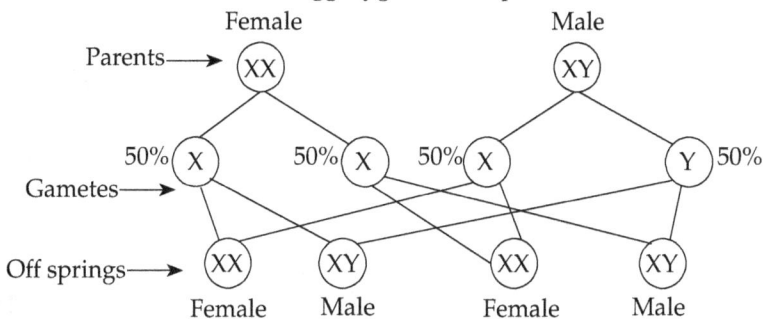

Sex determination in human

Sometime sex determination is regulated by environmental factor. In some reptiles temperature determine the sex at which the fertilized egg is incubated.

In human each cell contains 46 chromosomes. Any addition or removal in the number of sex chromosome or autosome cause genetic disorder.

1. **Klinefelter Syndrome:** When a male have an extra X or Y chromosome in sex chromosome then the condition will'be XXY or XYY instead of XY. The individual with, this syndrome have masculine development but feminine development is not completely suppressed and the individual became sterile.

In female when extra X chromosome is present instead of XX they show normal development but limited fertility. Mental retardness is also seen in this type of syndrome, Number of chromosome became 47 instead of 46.

2. **Turner's Syndrome :** When female has single sex chromosome (X0) their ovaries are rudimentary, lack of secondary sexual character.

3. **Down's Syndrome :** When an extra chromosome is added to 21st autosomal chromosomes this lead to develop Down's syndrome. In this syndrome person became Mangolism. The person is mentally retarded, eyes protruded an irregular physical structure is present.

4. **Patau's Syndrome :** This type of syndrome is develop by an addition of autosomal chromosome in 13th chromosome. There is a cut mark in the lip and person is mentally retarded. Diseases due to change in gentical constituent of chromosome.

1. **Sickle Cell Anaemia :** In this disorder erythrocytes destroyed more rapidly than normal leading to anaemia. These occur due to change in 11th autosomal chromosome.

2. **Phenylketonuria:** It is an inborn error of metabolism which result in mental retardation cause due to change in 12th autosomal chromosomes.

3. **Haemophilia :** Gene responsible for this disorder is linked with sex chromosomes. This disease lead to failure of blood clotting.

4. **Colour blindness :** This disorder lead to failure to distinugished red & green colour. The gene responsible for this disease is situated on sex chromosomes.

Number of Chromosomes in Different Organisms:

Pigeon	80	Dog	78	Horse	64
Chimpanz	48	Patato	48	Human	46
Rabbit	44	Wheat	42	Cat	38
Frog	26	Tamato	24	Pea	14
House-fly	12	Mosquito	6	Ascaris	2

7. Organic Evolution

More and more creation of organism by gradual changes from low categories animal to higher animal is called *organic evolution*. There are several evidence regarding organic evolution.

➪ **Homologous organ:** Organ which are seen different due to use in various function but its structure and embryonic development are similar. Ex — *Flipper of whale, feather of bat, forelimb of horse, Paw of cat,* and *hands of human.*

➪ **Analogous organ :** Organ which looks similar due to be used in similar function but their internal structure and embryonic development are different. Ex — *Feather of butterfly, bats* and *birds* all *looks* similar but their internal structure and origin are different.

➪ **Vestigial organ :** These are organs which appear functionless in an organism but functional in their ancestor. For example *vermiform appendix of large intestine and nictitating membrane of human.* Vermiform appendix is functional in herbivorous mammal even now.

- ⇨ **Fossils :** Fossils are the remains of ancient plant or animal which provide evidences for evolution. Example — Archaeoptery.
- ⇨ **Archaeopteryx :** It is a fossils look like bird but bear a number of features found in reptiles. So, it is a connecting link between aves and reptile.

Theories of Evolution

1. **Carolus Linnaeus** (1707–1778) contribution to classification provide an evolutionary relationship among the organism. He was also supported an idea that no species is new. Each and every species originates from some pre-existing species.

2. **Jean Baptist Lamarck** (1744 –1829) tried to explain the evolutionary process in his book *Philosophic zoologique*. The theory proposed by Lamark is known as *theory of inheritance of acquired characters*. According to this theory use and disuse of an organ lead to acquiring change in the features of that organ. These changes are also inherited to offspring. The favourable changes after long period of time result in evolution of new species. But *Lamarckism* was very strongly criticised by *August Weismann*.

3. **Charles Robert Darwin** (1809 – 1882) explain the evolutionary principle in his book *'The origin of species'*. The theory proposed by him is popularly known as *'Theory of natural selection' or Darwinism*. Darwin explained that despite having the enormous potential of fertility, the population of organism remains within a limit. It is due to struggle between members of same species and different species for food, space and mate. Struggle eliminates the unfit individual. The fit organism possess some variations which are favourable and they can leave the progeny to continue the favourable variation. The variation when accumalated for long time give rise to origin of new species with progress in genetics, the sources of variation were explained and Darwin's theory was modified. Now the most excepted theory of evolution is *Modern synthetic theory*, in which origin of species is based on the interaction of genetic variation and natural selection.

Botany

The study of different types of Trees, plants is called *Botany*.
Theophrastus is called the *father of Botany*.

1. Classification of Plantae

⇨ In the year 1883, **Eichler** has classified the Botanical world as under:

Plant Kingdom

```
                              Plant Kingdom
                                   |
           ┌───────────────────────┴───────────────────────┐
           ▼                                                 ▼
      Cryptogames                                      Phanerogames
   (Plant without seed)                              (Seed bearing plant)
           |                                                 |
    ┌──────┼──────────┐                         ┌────────────┴────────────┐
    ▼      ▼          ▼                         ▼                         ▼
Thalophyta  Bryophyta  Pteridophyta         Gymnospermae            Angiospermae
    |                                                        ┌───────────┴──────────┐
 ┌──┴────┐                                                   ▼                      ▼
 ▼       ▼                                            Monocotyledons          Dicotyledons
Thalophyta  Bryophyta
```

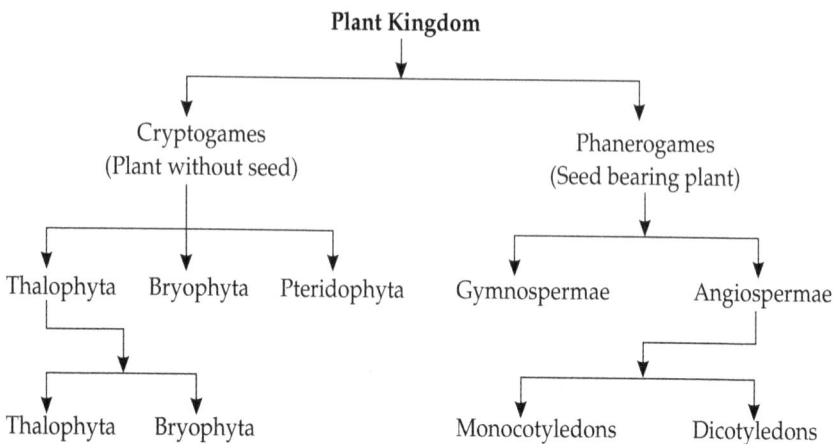

I. Cryptogamus plants

There is no flower and seed in these type of plants. These are classified into the following groups:

Thalophyta :

1. This is the largest group of the plant kingdom.
2. The body of the plants in this group is thalus like i.e., plant are not differentiated into root, stem and leaves etc.
3. There is no conducting tissue. It is divided into two groups.
   (a) Algae and (b) Fungi

(a) Algae

1. The study of algae is called *Phycology*.
2. The algae normally have *chlorophyll* and *autrotrophic* mode of nutrition.
3. Its body is thalus like. It may be *unicellular, colonial* or *filamentous*.

Useful Algae :

1. As a food : *Porphyra, Ulva, Surgassum, Laeminaria, Nostoc* etc.
2. In making Iodine : *Laeminaria, Pucus, Echlonia* etc.
3. As a manure : *Nostoc, Anabina, kelp* etc.
4. In making medicines : *Chloreloline* from *Chlorella* and *Tincher iodine* is made from *Laminaria*.
5. In research works : *Chlorella Acitabularia, Belonia* etc.

Note : *An astronaut can get protein food, water and oxygen by sowing the chlorella algae in the tank of the aircraft so chlorella is known as space algae.*

(b) Fungi

1. Study of fungi is called *Mycology*.

2. Fungi is chlorophyll less, central carrier tissue less, Thalophyte.
3. Accumulated food in fungi remains as *Glycogen*.
4. Its cell wall is made up of *chitin*. Ex. Albugo, Phytophthora Mucor etc.

Fungi may creates serious diseases in plants. Most damage is caused by rust and smut. Main Fungal diseases in plants are as :

White rust of crucifer, Loose smut of wheat, Rust of wheat, early Blight of potato, Red rot of sugarcane, Tikka diseases of ground nut, Wart disease of potato, Brown leaf spot of rice, Late blight of potato, Damping off of *seedlings* etc.

Bryophyta

This is the first group of land plants. In this division approximately 25000 species are included.

1. In byophyta there is lack of Xylem and phloem tissue.
2. Plant body may be of thallus like and leafy erect structure as in moss.
3. They lack true roots, Stem and leaves.
4. This community is also called *Amphibian category of the plant kingdom*.

The moss namely Sphagnum is capable of soaking water 18 times of its own weight. Therefore, gardeners use it to protect from drying while taking the plants from one place to another.

The Sphagnum moss is used as fuel.

The Sphagnum moss is also used as antiseptic.

Pteridophyta

The plants of this group are mostly found in wet shady places, forests and mountains.

1. The body of plants are differentiated into root, stem, and leaves. Stem remains as normal rhizome.
2. Reproduction occurs by spores produced inside the sporangia.
3. Gametophytic phase is short lived. The diploid zygote develops into an embryo.
4. Plants of this community have conducting tissues. But Xylem does not contain Vessels and Phloem does not contain companion cells.
   Examples : Ferns, Azolla, Pteridium, Lycopodium etc.

II. Phanerogamus or Floral plant

The plants in this group are well developed. All the plants in this group have flowers, fruits and seeds. The plants in this group can be classified into two sub-groups — *Gymnosperm* and *Angiosperm*.

(A) Gymnosperm

1. These plants are in the forms of trees and bushes. Plant body are differentiated into root, stem & leaves.
2. Plants are woody, perennial and tall. Plant bear naked seed.
3. Its tap roots are well developed.
4. Pollination takes place through air.

The longest plant of the Plant kingdom, *Sequoia gigentia* comes under it. Its height is 120 meters. This is also called *Red Wood of California*.
⇨ The smallest plant is *Zaimia Pygmia*.
⇨ Living fossils are *Cycas, Ginkgo, biloba* and *Metasequoia*.
⇨ *Ginkgo biloba* is also called *Maiden hair tree*.
⇨ Ovules and Antherzoids of *Cycas* is the largest in Plant kingdom.

The pollen grains of Pinus are so much in number that later it turns into Sulphur showers.

Importance of Gymnosperm
1. *As a food* – Sago is made by extracting the juice from the stems of Cycas. Therefore, Cycas is called *Sago-palm*.
2. *Wood*– The wood of Pine, Sequoia, Deodar, Spruce etc. is used for making furniture.
3. *Vapour oil* – We get Tarpin oil from the trees of Pine, Cedrus oil from Deodar tree and Cedcast oil from Juniperous wood.
4. *Tannin* – It is useful in tanning and making ink.
5. *Resin* – Resin is extracted from some conical plants which are used in making varnish, polish, paint etc.

(B) Angiosperm
1. In the plants of this sub-group seeds are found inside the fruits.
2. In there plants root, leaves, flowers, fruits and seeds are fully developed.

In the plants of this sub-group there is seed-coat in seeds. On the basis of number of cotyledons plants are divided into two categories –

1. *Monocotyledon* and (2) *Dicotyledon*

Monocotyledon plants : Those plants which have only one cotyledon in seed. Example :

	Name of category	Name of main plants
1.	*Liliaceae*	Garlic, Onion etc.
2.	*Palmae*	Nut, Palm, Coconut, Date etc.
3.	*Graminaeceae*	Wheat, Maize, Bamboo, Sugarcane, Rice, Bajra Oat etc.

Dicotyledons plants : Those plants which have two cotyledon in its seed are called *dicotyledons*. Example :

	Name of category	Name of main plants
1.	*Cruciferae*	Radish, Turnip, Mustard etc.
2.	*Malvaceae*	Jute, Lady's finger.
3.	*Leguminaceae*	Babool, Lajwanti, Ashok, Tamarind and all the Pulse crops.
4.	*Composite*	Sunflower, Marigold, Lily etc.
5.	*Rutaceae*	Lemon, Orange etc.
6.	*Cucurbitaceae*	Melon, Water melon, Guard, Bitter etc.
7.	*Solanaceae*	Potato, Chilly, Brinjal, Belladonna, Tomato etc.
8.	*Rosaceae*	Strawberry, Apple, Almond etc.

Virus

⇨ Study of virus is virology.

⇨ Virus was discovered by Russian scientist *Ivanovsky* in the year 1892. (During the tests of Mosaic disease on tobacco).

⇨ In nature, there are ultra microscopic particle known as viruses. Virus are connecting a link between living & non-living.

⇨ It has both the characters of living and non-living, so it is a connecting link between living & non-living.

Characters of virus

1. They became active inside a living cells.
2. Nucleic acids replicate themselves and they reproduce rapidly.
3. They cause disease like bacteria & fungi.

According to parasitic nature, virus is of three types –

1. *Plant virus* – RNA is present as its nucleic acid.
2. *Animal virus* – DNA or sometimes RNA is found in it.
3. *Bacteriophage* – They depend only on bacteria. They kill the bacteria. DNA is found in them. *Example* – T-2 phage.

⇨ In man virus cause disease like mumps, chicken pox, hepatitis, palio, AIDs and Herpes.

⇨ **Bacteriophages :** Bacteriophages are those virus which infect the bacteria Example —Tobacco mosaic virus.

Note : *Those viruses in which RNA substance is found as genetic material are called Retrovirus.*

Bacteria

It was discovered by *Antony von Lecuwenhoek* of Holland in the year 1683.

⇨ *Lecuwenhoek* is called the *father of Bacteriology*.

In the year 1829 *Ehrenberg* called it bacteria.

⇨ The year 1843-1892 – Robert Koch discovered the bacteria of Tuberculosis diseases.

⇨ The year 1812-1892 – *Louis Pasteur* discovered the vaccine of Rabies and pasteurization of milk.

⇨ On the basis of shape, bacteria is of different types :

1. **Bacillus :** This is rod-like or cylindrical.

2. **Round or Cocus :** These are round and the smallest bacteria.

3. **Comma shaped or Vibrio:** Like the English sign (,), example - *Vibrio cholerae* etc.

4. **Spirillum :** Spring or screw shaped.

⇨ Some species of *Azotobacter, Azospirillum* and *Clostridium* bacteria live freely in the soil and fix atmospheric nitrogen into the nitrogenous compound.

Anabaena and *Nostoc cynobacteria* fix atmospheric nitrogen into soil.

⇨ The species of *Rhizobium* and *Bradyrhizobium* etc. bacteria live in the roots of the Leguminous plants capable of converting atmospheric nitrogen into its compound.

Note : *To preserve the milk for many days pasteurization is done. There are two methods of pasteurization —*

    (a) **Low temperature holding method (LTH) :** *Milk is boiled at 62.8°C for 30 minutes.*

    (b) **High Temperature short time method (HTSt):** *Milk is boiled at 71.7°C for 15 seconds.*

⇨ In leather industry separation of hair and fat from leather is done by bacteria. This is called *tanning of leather.*

⇨ Pickles, syrup is kept in salt or in dense liquid of sugar so that in case of bacterial attack bacteria are plasmolysed and destroyed. Therefore, pickles etc. do not get spoiled soon and can be preserved for long time.

⇨ In the Cold Storage objects are kept at low temperature (-10°C to -18°C).

⇨ **Mycoplasma :** Smallest known prokaryotic cell *pleuropneumonia*. It is also known as PPLO.

2. Plant Morphology

Morphology : The study of forms and features of different parts of plants like roots, stems, leaves, flowers, fruits etc. is called Morphology.

Root

Root is the descending part of the plant which develops from *radicle*.

Root always grows in the soil away from light.

Roots are of two types—

(i) *Tap root* and   (ii) *Adventitious root*

Modification of Tap roots are :

1. *Conical* – like carrot   2. *Napiform* – like Turnip, beet etc.

3. *Fusiform* – like radish.

Stem

This is the part of a plant which grows towards light.

It develops from *plumule*.

The modification of stems are as under–

Underground stem

1. *Tuber* – like Potato.   2. *Corm* – like Colocasia, Saffron etc.

3. *Bulb* – like Onion, Garlic etc.   4. *Rhizome* – like Turmeric, Ginger etc.

Leaf

It is green. Its main function is to make food through photosynthesis.

Flower

This is the reproductive part of the plant.

In the flower *Calyx, Corolla, Androecium* and *Gynoecium* are found. Out of these androecium is male sex organ and the Gynoecium is female sex organ.

↪ **Androecium :** Unit of androcium is stamen there is one or more stamens in the androecium. Pollen grains are found in another.

↪ **Gynoecium :** Unit of gynoecium is *carpel*. There are three parts of carpel – (i) *Ovary*, (ii) *Style* and (iii) *Stigma*.

↪ **Pollination :** After maturation of Anther, the process of reaching of pollen grains to stigma is called *pollination*. Pollination is of two types– (i) *Self-pollination*   (ii) *Cross-pollination*

↪ **Fertilization :** Pollen tube reaches the egg cell after entering into the ovule through a pore called *micryopyle*. After that a male nucleus fuse with egg-cell. This is called *fertilization*. Fertilized egg is called *zygote*.

In angiosperm, the fertilization is triple fusion whereas in other category of plants it is double fusion.

↪ **Parthenocarpy :** In some plants fruits are developed from ovary without fertilization. This type of fruit is called *parthenocarpy*. Normally these types of fruits are seedless. ***Example–*** Banana, Papaya, Orange, Grapes, Pine-apple etc.

Formation of fruits

Fruit is a matured or ripened ovary developed after fertilization.

Formation of fruit takes place from ovary. Fruits are divided into three types-

1. *Simple fruits–* like Banana, Guava etc.
2. *Aggregate fruit–* Strawberry, Custard apple etc.
3. *Composite fruit–* Jackfruit, Mulbery etc.

In the development of some fruits, Calyx, Corolla and thalmus takes part. These types of fruits are called *False fruits*. ***Example–*** Apple, Jackfruit, pear etc.

Some Fruits and Their Edible Parts

Fruit	Edible part	Fruit	Edible part
Apple	Fleshy thalamus	*Wheat*	starchy endosperm
Pear	Fleshy thalamus	*Cashew nut*	Peduncle & cotyledons
Mango	Mesocarp	*Lichi*	Aril
Guava	Entire fruit	*Gram*	cotyledons & embryo
Grapes	Pericarp and Placenta	*Groundnut*	Cotyledons
Papaya	Mesocarp	*Mulberry*	entire fruit
Coconut	Endosperm	*Jackfruit*	Bract, Perianth and seed
Tomato	Pericarp and Placenta	*Pine apple*	Bract and Perianth
Banana	Mesocarp & Endocarp	*Orange*	Juicy hair

3. Plant Tissue

Tissue : The group of cells of similar origin, structure and functions is called tissue.

Types of Plant Tissue

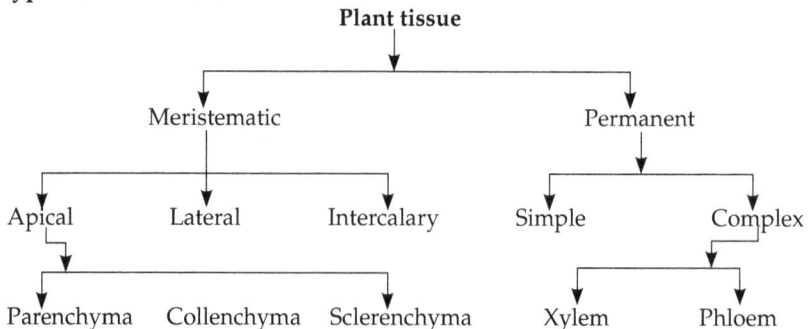

(A) Meristematic tissue : Growing regions of the plants are called *Meristem*. Meristematic tissue have capability of cell division. Daughter cells formed out. It grow and constitute the different parts of the plant. This process continues till the life-span of the plant.

Specific features of the Meristematic tissues are as follows :

(i)   It is round, oval or multi-sided.

(ii) Its wall is thin and cytoplasm is homogeneous.

(iii) Cell contains dense cytoplasm and a single large nucleus.

(iv) There is lack of inter-cellular spaces between the cells.

⇨ **Apical Meristems :** These tissues are found in the root and stem apex and the initial growth (specially length) of the plants take place due to these tissue.

⇨ **Lateral Meristems :** Due to the division in these tissue growth in the girth of roots and stems takes place. Hence, it increases the width of the root and stem.

⇨ **Intercalary Meristems :** They are located at the base of internode. In fact, this is the remains of the Apical Meristems, which is divided by the incoming of permanent tissues in the centre. Plants increase its length by the activity of this. Its importance is for those plants whose apex parts are eaten by vegetarian animals. After peing eaten the apex part the plants grow with the help of intercalary meristems only. Like – grass.

(B) Permanent tissue : Permanent tissues are made of those mature tissues that have lost their capacity of division and attain a definite forms for various works. These cells can be alive or dead.

⇨ **Simple tissue :** If permanent tissue is made up of similar types of cells, it is called *simple tissue*.

⇨ **Complex tissue :** If permanent tissue is made up of one or more types of cells, it is called *Complex tissue*.

⇨ **Xylem:** This is usually called *wood*. This is conducting tissue. Its two main functions are–

(i)   Conduction of water and minerals and

(ii) To provide mechanical consistency.

The determination of age of the plant is done by counting annual rings of the xylem tissue. The method of determining the age of plant is called Dendrochronology.

⇨ **Phloem :** This is a conducting tissue. Its main function is to conduct foods prepared by the leaves to different parts of the plant.

4. Photosynthesis

In the presence of water, light, chlorophyll and carbon dioxide, the formation of carbohydrates in plant is called *photosynthesis*.

$$6CO_2 + 12H_2O \xrightarrow[\text{Chlorophyll}]{\text{Light}} C_6H_{12}O_6 + 6H_2O + 6O_2$$

Clucose   Water   Oxygen

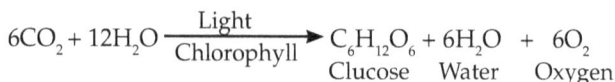

Carbon dioxide, water, chlorophyll and sunlight are necessary for photosynthesis.

⇨ Terrestrial plants takes CO_2 from atmosphere whereas aquatic plants use carbon dioxide mixed in water.

⇨ Water enters into the cells of the leaves through osmosis and CO_2 through diffusion from atmosphere or release during respiration.

⇨ Water necessary for photosynthesis is absorbed by the roots and the oxygen produced during photosynthesis is due to photolysis of water.

⇨ The green colour of the plants is due to the presence of chlorophyll. Chlorophyll are photoreceptor molecule, which trap the solar energy. There are different type of chlorophyll molecule like 'a', 'b', 'c', 'd' & 'e'. Chlorophyll 'a' & 'b' are most common and are found in a plant.

⇨ There is an atom of magnesium in the centre of chlorophyll.

⇨ Chlorophyll absorbs the violet, blue and red colours of light.

The rate of photosynthesis is maximum in red light and is minimum in violet light.

⇨ The process of photosynthesis is a reaction of oxidation and reduction. Oxidation of water takes place forming oxygen and reduction of carbon dioxide takes place forming glucose.

The stages of process of photosynthesis

(i) Photochemical reaction or light reaction and

(ii) Dark chemical reaction

(i) **Photochemical reaction :** This reaction is completed in the grana part of the chlorophyll. This is also called *Hill reaction*. In this process break down of water takes place and hydrogen ion and electron is formed. For photolysis of water, energy is received from the light. At the end of this process, ATP is formed from ADP & P.

(ii) **Dark chemical reaction :** This reaction takes place in the stroma of chlorophyll. In this reaction reduction of carbon dioxide takes place and sugar or starch are formed. It is also known as *Calvin Benson cycle*.

5. Plant Hormones

Following five hormones are found in plants –

1. **Auxins :** Auxins was discovered by Darwin in the year 1880.

   This is the hormone which controls the growth of plants.

   Its formation takes place in the apex parts of the plants.

   Its main functions are –

(i)   It prevents the separation of the leaves.

(ii) It destroys the straws.

(iii) It saves the crops from falling.

2. **Gibberellins:** It was discovered by a Japanese scientist *Kurosava* in the year 1926.

Functions:

(i)   It turns the dwarf plants into long plants. It helps in creating flowering.

(ii) It hep in breaking the dormancy of plant.

(iii) It motivates the seeds to be sprout.

(iv) It increases the activity of cambium in the wooden plants.

(v)   Large sized fruits and flowers can be produced by its scattering.

3. **Cytokinins:** It was discovered by z in the year 1955 but it was named byLethem.

Functions:

(i)   It naturally works in coordination with auxins.

(ii) It help in cell division and development in the presence of auxins.

(iii) It help in breaking the dormancy of seed.

(iv) It is helpful in making RNA and protein.

4. **Abscisic Acid or ABA** : This hormone was initially discovered by Carnes and Adicote and later on by *Waring*.

Functions:

(i)   This hormone is against the growth.

(ii) It keeps the seeds & bud in dormant condition.

(iii) It plays main role in separation of leaves.

(iv) It delays in flowering of long day plant.

5. **Ethylene** : This is the only hormone which is found in gaseous form.

Functions:

(i)   It helps in the ripening the fruits.

(ii) It increases the number of female flowers.

(iii) It motivates the separation of leaves, flowers and fruits.

6. **Florigens** : It is formed in leaves but helps in blooming of the flowers. Therefore, it is also called *flowering hormones*.

7. **Traumatic** : This is a type of dicarboxylic acid. It is formed in injured cells by which the injury of plants is healed.

6. Plant Diseases

1. **Viral Diseases :**
   (i) *Mosaic disease of tobacco* – In this disease leaves get shrinked and become small. The chlorophyll of leaves get destroyed. The factor of this disease is *Tobacco Mosaic Virus* (TMV).
   Control – Affected plants should be burnt.
   (ii) *Bunchy top of banana* – This diseases is caused by *banana virus*. In this disease plants become dwarf and all the leaves get accumulated like a rose on the branch.

2. **Bacterial Disease :**
   (i) **Wilt of Potato** : It is also known as ring *disease* because brown ring is formed on the xylem. The factor of this disease is *Pseudomonas solonacearum* bacteria. In this disease the conduction system of the plant is affected.
   (ii) **Black Arm of cotton** : The factor of this disease is *Xanthomonas Bacteria*. In this disease a water body (brown) is formed on the leaves.
   (iii) **Bacterial blight of Rice** : This disease is caused by *Xanthomonas oryzae bacteria*. Yellow-greenish spot is seen on both sides of leaves. Vascular bundles get blocked due to bacterial growth.

   (iv) **Citrus Canker** : The factor of this disease is *Xanthomonas citri* bacteria. It has originated in China. Leaves, branches, fruits all are affected by this disease.
   (v) **Tundu disease of wheat** : The factors of this disease are *Corinobacterium titrici* bacteria and Enzuina Titriki Nematode. In this disease lower parts of the leaves are faded and turned.

3. **Fungal Diseases :** The diseases included in this group are caused by fungi.

Some Important Facts Regarding Botany

Facts	Example and details
Largest angiosperm tree	*Eucalyptus*
Longest tree in the world	*Sequoia* giganteum. This is a gymnosperm. Its height is 120 meter. This is also called *Coast Red Wood of California.*
Smallest(in shape) angiosperm plant	Lemna. This is aquatic angiosperm which is found in India too.
Plant with largest leaf	Victoria Regia. This is an aquatic plant which is found in West Bengal in India.

Largest fruit	*Lodoicea* . This is also called double coconut. This is found in Kerala in India.
Smallest Pteridophyta	*Azolla*. This is an aquatic plant.
Smallest seed	*Orchid*
Smallest flower	*Wolfia*. Its diameter is 0.1 millimeter.
Largest flower	*Reflesia arnoldii*. Its diameter is 1 meter and its weight can be 8 kilograms.
Smallest angiosperm parasite	*Arceuthobium* is a parasite on the stems of gymnosperms.
Largest male couplet	*Cycas*. This is a gymnosperm plant.
Largest seed-egg	*Cycas*
Alivemorph	*Cycas*
Smallest chromosomes	*In algae*
Longest chromosomes	*In Trillium*
The plant with the largest number of Chromosomes	Ophioglossum *(Fern)*. There are 1266 chromosomes in its Diploid cell.
The plant with the least number of chromosomes	Heplapapopus *gracilis*.
The smallest gymnosperm	*Zamia pygmea*
The heaviest wooden plant	*Hardwichia binata*.
The lightest wooden plant	*Ochroma lagopus-balsa*
The smallest cell	*Mycoplasma gallisepticum*
Fruit like a tenills ball	*Kenth*
Fire of the forest	*Dhak*
Coffee giving plant	*Coffea arabica*. Caffin contains in it.
Coco giving plant	*Theobroma cococa*. Theobromin and caffeine contain in it.
Caffeine	*Pepaver somniferum* morphin contains in it.

7. Ecology

⇨ Study of inter relationship between living organisms and their environment.

⇨ Various population of living in a definite place is called *Biotic Community*.

⇨ Ecosystem or Ecological system word was first coined by the scientist namely *Tansley*.

Every ecosystem is made up of two components –

(a) Biotic component – Living part
(b) Abiotic component – Non living part

(a) Biotic components : It is divided into three parts –
(1) Producer (2) Consumer (3) Decomposers

(1) Producer : Those components that make their own food. Like – green plants.

(2) Consumer : Those components that consumes the food made by plant. Consumers are of three types:

(i) *Primary consumers :* In this category those organisms are included that lives on green plants or some parts of them.

(ii) *Secondary consumers :* In this category those organisms are included that depends on the primary consumers as their food. Like – fox, wolf, peacock etc.

(iii) *Tertiary consumers :* In this category those organisms are included that depends on the secondary consumers. Like – Tiger, lion, cheetah etc.

(3) Decomposers : Mainly fungi and bacteria are included in this category. These decomposes dead producers and consumers and changes them into physical elements.

(b) Abiotic components : Abiotic components are as follows:

(i) Carbonic substance, (ii) Non-carbonic substance, (iii) Climatic factor

Example : Water, light, temperature, air, humidity, minerals etc.

⇨ **Food Chain :** Transfer of energy from the producer through a series of organisms.

8. Nitrogen Cycle

⇨ Nitrogen fixation is a process in which free atmosphberic nitrogen is converted by living organism into nitrogenous compound that can be used by plant.

⇨ **Ammonification :** Formation of ammonia from organic compound like proteins and nucleic acid by microorganism.

⇨ **Nitrification :** A process in which ammonia is converted into nitrates and nitrates by Nitrobacteria.

⇨ **Denitrification :** It is the process of converting fix nitrogen like nitrates, nitrites and ammonia into free nitrogen by denitrifying bacteria eg Pseudonymouna.

9. Pollution

Unwanted changes in the chemical and physical features of air, water and land (environment) that are dangerous to human and other organisms, their life conditions, industrial process and cultural achievements are called *pollution.*

The types of pollution are mainly —(i) Air pollution, (ii) Water pollution, (iii) Sound pollution, (iv) Soil pollution, (v) Nuclear pollution.

(i) **Air pollution :** When the pollution is in the atmosphere and the sufficient quantity of atmosphere reduces then it is called *Air pollution.*

Main air pollutants — *Carbon monoxide* (CO), Sulphur dioxide (SO_2), Hydrogen sulphide (H_2S), Hydrogen fluoride (HF), Nitrogen oxide (NO and NO_2), Hydrocarbon, Ammonia (NH_3), Smoke of tobacco, Fluorides smoke and particles of smoke, Aerosols etc.

Sulphur dioxide (SO_2), Sulphur trioxide (SO_3), Nitrogen oxide (NO) react with environmental water and creates Sulphuric acid and Nitric acid. These acids reach the earth with rain water and this is called *acid rain.*

On 3rd December, 1984 an incidence of leakage of Methyl Isocyanide gas took place in the fertilizer making Union Carbide Factory. (Bhopal)

(ii) **Water pollution :** Mixing of unwanted substances with water is called *water pollution.*

Sources of water pollution : The water pollution takes place mainly due to mixing up of Carbonate, sulphates of Magnesium and Potassium, Ammonia, Carbon monoxide, Carbon dioxide and Industrial remains in water. Sea-water pollution is due to mixing up of heavy metals, hydro carbon, petroleum etc. in water.

(iii) **Sound pollution:** The unwanted and undesirable sounds scattered in atmosphere are called *sound pollution.*

Sources of sound pollution : The source of sound pollution is loud sound or noise, in whatever ways it has produced.

(iv) **Soil pollution :** Distorted form of soil is called *Soil pollution.*

Sources of Soil pollution: acid rain, water from mines, excessive use of fertilizers and germicide chemicals, garbage, industrial remainins, excretion in open field etc. are the main sources of soil pollution.

(v) **Nuclear pollution :** This pollution is created by radioactive rays.

Following can be the sources of radioactive pollution –

(i) Pollution from the rays which are used in treatment.

(ii) Pollution created from fuels used in atomic reactors.

(iii) Pollution created from the use of nuclear weapons.

(iv) Pollution created remaining substances coming out of Atomic power-houses.

Population, Biotic Community

⇨ **Population** : Population is a group of individuals of same species occupying the same area at a given time.

⇨ **Population density** : Total number of individual present in per unit area.

⇨ **Natality** : Increase in the number of individuals in a given population by birth is called natality.

⇨ **Mortality** : Number of individuals removed from a population due to death under given environmental condition at a given time is called mortality.

⇨ **Biotic potential** : It refers the maximum capacity of inherent of an organism to reproduce.

⇨ **Environmental resistance** : Environmental factors, which put a check on the growth of population.

⇨ **Mutalism** : It is a functional association between two different species in which both the species are benefited.

⇨ **Commensalism:** It is an association between individuals of two different species in which one species is benefited and other one is neither benefited nor affected.

⇨ **Population Explosion** : The dramatic increase in population size over a relatively short period is called population explosion.

⇨ **Demographic transition:** If the birth rate is equal to the death rate, it results in zero population growth, which is called demographic transition.

⇨ **Psychosis** : It is a mild form of mental illness where the patient show prolonged emotional reaction.

⇨ **Drug abuse:** When drugs are taken for a purpose other than their normal clinical use in an amount that impairs ones physical, physiological and psychological function of body is called drug abuse.

Zoology

Zoology : Scientific study of the structure, form and distribution of animals.

1. Classification of Animal Kingdom

Animals kingdom of the world is divided into two sub-kingdoms :

(i) Unicellular animal   (ii) Multi-cellular animal.

Unicellular animals are kept in a single phylum Protozoa whereas multi-cellular animals are divided into 9 phylums.

Classification of animals according to *Storer* and *Usinger*–

A. **Phylum Protozoa : Main features** – Unicellular
   (i) It's body is made of only one cell.
   (ii) There is one or more nuclei in its cytoplasm.
   (iii) Are both the types commensalism and parasite.
   (iv) All the metabolic activity (eating, digestion, respiration, excretion, reproduction) takes place in unicellular body.
   (v) Respiration and excretion take place by diffusion.
   Example – *Amoeba, Euglena, Trypanosoma* etc.

B. **Phylum Porifera :** All animal of this group are found in marine water & bear pores in body.
   (i) These are multicellular animals but cells do not make regular tissues.
   (ii) Numerous pores known as *ostia* found on body wall.
   (iii) Skeleton is made up of minute calcareous or silicon spicules.
   Example – *Sycon, Sponge* etc.

C. **Phylum Coelenterate : Main features** – Coelenteron is present
   (i) Animals are aquatic and diploblastic.
   (ii) Around the mouth some thread-like structure are found known as tentacles, which help in holding the food.
   (iii) Body radial symmetry.
   (iv) Specialized cnidoblast cell are found help in catching the food.
   Example – *Hydra, Jelly fish, Sea Anemone* etc.

D. **Phylum Platyhelminthes : Main features** – Flat worm
   (i) Triploblastic and no body cavity.
   (ii) Dorso-ventraly flattened animal.
   (iii) Alimentary canal with single opening, anus absent.
   (iv) Excretion takes place by flame cells.
   (v) There is no skeleton, respiratory organ, circulatory system etc.
   (vi) These are hermaphrodite animal.
   Example – *Planaria, Liver fluke, Tape worm* etc.

E. **Phylum Ascheleminthes : Main features** – Round worm
   (i) Long, cylindrical, unsegmented worm.
   (ii) Bilaterally symmetrical and triploblastic.
   (iii) Alimentary canal is complete in which mouth and anus both are present.

(iv) There is no circulatory & respiratory systems but nervous system is developed.

(v) Excretion takes place through *Protonephridia*.

(vi) They are unisexual.

(vii) Most form are parasitic but some are free living in soil & water.

Example – Round worm, like – *Ascaris, Thread worm, Wuchereia* etc.

Note : *(i) Enterobius (pin worm/thread worm) – It is found mainly in the anus of child. Children feel itching and often vomits. Some children urinate on the bed at night.*

(ii) Filarial disease is caused by Wuchereia bancrofti.

F. **Phylum Annelida : Main features –** Annulus body Bearing ring

(i) Body is long, thin, soft and metamerically segmented.

(ii) Locomotion takes place through *Setae* made up of Chitin.

(iii) Alimentary canal is well developed.

(iv) Normally respiration through skin, in some animals it takes place through *coelom*.

(v) Nervous system is normal and blood is red.

(vi) Excretion by *nephridia*.

(vii) Both unisexual and bisexual.

Example – *Earthworm, Nereis, Leech* etc.

Note : *There are four pairs of heart in earthworm.*

G. **Phylum Arthropoda : Main features –** Jointed leg

(i) Body is divided into three parts - Head, Thorax and Abdomen.

(ii) Body is covered with a thick chitinous exoskeleton.

(iii) Jointed leg.

(iv) Circulatory system is open type.

(v) Its body cavitys are called *haemocoel*.

(vi) *Trachea, book lungs, body surface* are respiratory parts.

(vii) These are mainly unisexual and fertilization takes place inside the body.

Example — *Cockroach, prawn, crab, bug, fly, mosquito, bees* etc.

Note : *(i) There are six feet and four wings in insects, (ii) There are 13 chamber in the Cockroach's heart, (iii) Ant is a social animal which reflects labour division, (iv) Termite is also a social animal which lives in colony.*

H. **Phylum Mollusca : Main features –** Soft bodies animal

(i) Body is soft divided into head and muscular foot.

(ii) Mantle is always present in it, which secretes a hard calcareous shell.

(iii) Alimentary canal is well developed.

(iv) Respiration takes place through *gills* or *ctenidia*.

(v) Blood is colourless.

(vi) Excretion takes place through kidneys.

Example – *Pila, Octopus, Loligo, Squid* etc.

Note :	Mollusca	Other name in vogue
	Aplysia	Sea rabbit
	Doris	Sea lemon
	Octopus	Devil-fish
	Sepia	Cuttle-fish

I. **Phylum Echinodermata : Main features** – Spiny skin

(i) All the animals in this group are marine.

(ii) Water vascular system is present.

(iii) There is Tube feet for locomotion, taking food which works as sensation organ.

(iv) Brain is not developed in nervous system.

(v) There is a special capacity of regeneration.

Example : *Star fish, Sea urchin, Sea cucumber, Brittle stars* etc.

Note : *The work of the Aristotle lantern is to chew the food. It is found in sea urchin.*

J. **Phylum Chordata : Main features**

(i) Notochord is present in it.

(ii) All the chordates are triploblastic, coelomate and bilaterally symmetrical.

(iii) A dorsal hollow tubular nerve cord and paired pharyngeal gill slits are other features of chordates.

According to classification there are two sub phyla in Chordata.

(a) Protochordates and (b) Vertebrata

Some main groups of phylum Chordata :

1. **Pisces : Main features** – Aquatic life

(i) All these are cold blooded animals.

(ii) Its heart pumps only impure blood and have two chamber.

(iii) Respiration takes place through *gills*.

Example : *Hippopotamus, Scoliodon, Torpedo*, etc.

2. **Amphibia : Main features** – Found both on land & water

(i) All these creatures are amphibian.

(ii) All these are cold-blooded.

(iii) Respiration takes place through gill, skin and lungs. Heart have three, chamber two auricles and one ventricle.

Example : Frog, Necturus, Toad, etc. *Icihyophis, Salamander.*

Note : *In fact the croaking of frogs is the call for sex.*

3. **Reptilia : Main features – Crawlling animal**

(i) Land vertebrate, cold-booded, terrestrial or aquatic vertebrates.

(ii) It contains two pair of limbs.

(iii) The skeleton is completely flexible.

(iv) Respiration takes place through lungs.

(v) Its eggs are covered with shell made up of Calcium carbonate.

Example : *Lizard, snake, tortoise, crocodile, turtle, sphenodon* etc.

Note : ✦ *Mesozoic era is called the era of reptiles.*

✦ *Cobra is the only snake which makes nests.*

✦ *Heloderma is the only poisonous lizard.*

✦ *Sea snake which is called Hydrophis is the world's most poisonous snake.*

4. **Aves : Main features** – Warm blooded tetrapod vertebrates with flight adaptation.

(i) Its fore-feet modified into wings to fly.

(ii) Boat shaped body is divisible into head , neck, trunk and tail.

(iii) Its respiratory organ is lungs.

(iv) Birds have no teeth, beak help in feeding.

Example : *crow, peacock, parrot* etc.

Note : *(i) Flightless Birds – Kiwi and Emus, (ii) Largest alive bird is Ostrich, (iii) Smallest bird is Humming bird, (iv) Largest zoo in India isAlipur (Kolkata) and the largest zoo of the world is Cruiser National Park in South Africa.*

5. **Mammalia : Main features**

(i) Sweat glands and oil glands are found on skin.

(ii) All these animals are warm blooded.

(iii) Its hearts are divided into four chamber.

(iv) Tooth comes twice in these animals. (Diphyodont)

(v) There is no nucleus in its red blood cells (except in camel and lama).

(vi) Skin of mammal have hair.

(vii) External ear is present.

Mammals are divided into three sub-classes :

(i) *Prototheria* - It lays eggs. Example - *Echidna.*

(ii) *Metatheria* - It bears the immature child. Example - Kangaroo,

(iii) *Eutheria* — It bears the well developed child. Example — *Human*.

Note : *(i) In mammal the highest body temperature is of goat. (Average 39 degree Celsius), (ii) Echidna and Duck billed Platypus are the egg laying mammal.*

2. Animal Tissue

The animal tissues can be divided into following categories-(i) Epithelial Tissue, (ii) Connective Tissue, (iii) Muscular Tissue, (iv) Nervous Tissue.

(i) **Epithelial Tissue :** Epithelial tissue cover the external surface of the body and internal free surface of many organs. Epithelial cell arranged very close to each other. There is no blood vessels supplying nourishment to epithelial cells. They receive nourishment from underlaying connective tissue. The principle functions of epithelial tissues are covering and lining of free surface.

Example— skin, intestine, gland, hollow organ like fallopian tube, nasal passage bronchioles, trachea etc.

(ii) **Connective Tissue :** These tissue connect and bind different tissues or organs. It provides the structural frame work and mechanical support to body. It play role in body as defense tissue, repair fat storage etc.

Example— Adipose tissue found beneath the skin. Ligament made up of fibrous connective tissue. Cartilage, bone and blood.

Note : *Blood is only tissue which is found in the form of fluid.*

⇨ (iii) **Muscular Tissue :** This is also known as contractile tissue. All the muscles of the body are made up of this tissue. Muscle tissue is of three types — (a) Unstriped, (b) Striped and (c) Cardiac

(a) **Unstriped :** This muscle tissue is found on the walls of those parts which do not controled by will. These are called involuntary muscle, like, Alimentary canal, Rectum, Ureter, Blood vessels. Unstriped muscles control the motions of all those organs that move on their own.

(b) **Striped :** These muscles are found in the parts of the body that move voluntary. Normally one or both the end of these muscles turn and connect with bones as tendon.

(c) **Cardiac :** These muscles are found only on the walls of the heart. The contraction and expansion of the heart is due to these muscles that move throughout the life without fail.

⇨ There are 639 muscles in the human body.

⇨ The largest muscle of the human body is *Gluteus Maximus* (muscle of the hip).

⇨ The smallest muscle of the human body is *Stapedius*.

(iv) Nervous Tissue : This tissue is also called sensitive tissue. The nervous systems of the organisms is made up of these tissues. This is made up of two specific cells - (a) Nerve cell or Neurons and (b) Neuroglia.

⇨ Nervous tissue controls all the voluntary & involuntary activities of the body.

3. Human Blood

⇨ Blood is a fluid connective tissue.

⇨ The quantity of blood in the human's body is 7% of the total weight.

⇨ This is a dissolution of base whose pH value is 7.4

⇨ There is an average of 5-6 litres of blood in human body.

⇨ Female contains half litre of blood less in comparison to male.

⇨ Blood is consist of two part—

(A) Plasma and (B) Blood corpuscles.

(A) Plasma : This is the liquid part of blood. 60% of the blood is plasma Its 90% parts is water, 7% protein, 0.9% salt and 0.1% is glucose. Remaining substances are in a very low quantity.

Function of plasma : Transportation of digested food, hormones, exeretory product etc. from the body takes place through plasma.

⇨ **Serum** : When Fibrinogen & protein is extracted out of plasma, the remaining plasma is called *serum*.

(B) Blood corpuscles : This is the remaining 40% part of the blood. This is divided into three parts -

(i) *Red Blood Corpuscles* (RBCs)

(ii) *White Blood Corpuscles* (WBCs) and (iii) *Blood Platelets*.

(i) Red Blood Corpuscles (RBC) : Red Blood Corpuscles (RBC) of a mammal is biconcave.

⇨ There is no nucleus in it. Exception - Camel and Lama.

RBC is formed in Bone marrow.

(At the embroynic stage its formation takes place in liver).

⇨ Its life span is from 20 days to 120 days.

⇨ Its destruction takes place in liver & spleen. Therefore, liver is called grave of RBC.

⇨ It contains haemoglobin, in which *haeme* iron containing compound is found and due to this the colour of blood is red.

⇨ *Globin* is a proteinous compound which is extremely capable of combining with oxygen and carbon dioxide.

⇨ The iron compound found in haemoglobin, is *haematin*.

⇨ The main function of RBC is to carry oxygen to all cells of the body and bring back the carbon dioxide.

➪ *Anaemia* disease is caused due the deficiency of haemoglobin.

➪ At the time of sleeping RBC reduced by 5% and people who are at the height of 4200 meters RBC increases by 30% in them.

(ii) White Blood Corpuscles (WBC) or Leucocytes : In shape and constitution this is similar to Amoeba.

➪ Its formation takes place in Bone marrow, lymph node and sometimes in liver and spleen.

➪ Its life span is from 1 to 2 days.

➪ Nucleus is present in the White Blood Corpuscles.

➪ Its main function is to protect the body from the disease.

➪ The ratio of RBC and WBC is 600 :1.

(iii) Blood Platelets or Thrombocytes : It is found only in the blood of human and other mammals.

➪ There is no nucleus in it.

➪ Its formation takes place in Bone marrow.

➪ Its life span is from 3 to 5 days.

➪ It dies in the Spleen.

➪ Its main function is to help in clotting of blood.

Functions of blood :

(i) To control the temperature of the body and to protect the body from diseases.

(ii) Clotting of blood.

(iii) Transportation of O_2, CO_2, digested food, conduction of hormones etc.

(iv) To help in establishing coordination among different parts.

Clotting of Blood : Three important reactions during clotting of blood.

(i) Thromboplastin + Prothrombin + Calcium = Thrombin.

(ii) Thrombin + Fibrinogen = Fibrin.

(iii) Fibrin + Blood Corpuscles = Clot.

The formation of Prothrombin and Fibrinogen of the blood plasma takes place with the help of Vitamin K. Vitamin K is helpful in making clots of blood. Normally clotting takes the time from 2 to 5 minutes.

The compulsory protein in making clots of blood is *Fibrinogen.*

Blood Group of human : Blood Group was discovered by Landsteiner in 1900. For this, he was awarded with Nobel Prize in the year 1930.

➪ The main reason behind the difference in blood of human is the glyco protein which is found in Red Blood Corpuscles called *antigen.*

Antigen are of two types – Antigen A and Antigen B.

➪ On the basis of presence of Antigen or Glyco Protein, there are four group of blood in human :

(a) That contains Antigen A - Blood Group A.

(b) That contains Antigen B - Blood Group B.

(c) That contains both the Antigens A and B - Blood Group AB.

(d) That contains neither of the Antigens - Blood Group O.

An opposite type of protein, is found in blood plasma. This is called *antibody*. This is also of two types – Antibody 'a' and Antibody 'b'.

⇨ Therefore, with the four groups of blood division of antibody is as under –

S.No.	Blood Group	Antigen (In Red Blood Corpuscles)	Antibody (In plasma)
1.	A	Only 'A'	Only 'b'
2.	B	Only 'B'	Only 'a'
3.	AB	Both 'A' and 'B'	Absent
4.	O	Absent	Both 'a' and 'b'

Blood Transfusion : Antigen 'A' and antibody 'a', Antigen 'B' and antibody 'b' cannot live together. In case of so happened these get most sticky, which spoils the blood. This is called *agglutination of blood*. Therefore, in blood transfusion adjustment of Antigen and Antibody should be done carefully so that agglutination of blood do not takes place.

Blood Group O is called Universal Donor because it does not contain any antigen.

Blood Group AB is called Universal Receptor because it does not contain any antibody.

Rh factor : In the year 1940, Landsteiner and Wiener discovered a different type of antigen in the blood. They discovered it in the *Rhesus monkey*, therefore, it is called *Rh-factor*. In the blood of that person it is found, their blood is called Rh-positive and in the blood of that person it is not found, is called *Rh-negative*.

At the time of blood transfusion Rh-factor is also tested. Rh+ is given to Rh+ and Rh⁻ is given Rh-blood only.

If the blood of Rh+ blood group is transmitted to a person with Rh⁻ blood group, then due to the less quantity for the first time there does not seem any bad effect but if this process is repeated then due to agglutination the person with Rh⁻ blood group dies.

Erythroblastosis Foetalis : If the father's blood is Rh+ and the mother's blood is Rh- then the child to be born dies at the pregnancy or short span of time after the birth. (This happens in the case of second issue).

The possible blood group of the child on the basis of blood group of mother and father.

Blood group of Mother and father	Expected blood group of the child	Unexpected blood of the child
O × O	O	A, B, AB
O × A	O, A	B, AB
O × B	O, B	A, AB
O × AB	A, B	O, AB
A × A	A, O	B, AB
A × B	O, A, B, AB	None
A × AB	A, B, AB	O
B × B	B, O	A, AB
B × AB	A, B, AB	O
AB × AB	A, B, AB	O

Haemolymph: Body fluid of arthropoda is a colourless made of plasma and haemocytes. It donot contain any respiratory pigment Ex—Cockroach.

4. System of the Human Body

(a) Digestive System

The complete process of nutritioin is divided into five stages :

1. Ingestion   2. Digestion   3. Absorption
4. Assimilation   5. Defecation

1. **Ingestion :** Taking the food into the mouth is called *Ingestion*.
2. **Digestion :** Conversion of nonabsorbable food into absorbable form. The digestion of the food is started from the mouth.

⇨ Saliva is secreted by salivary gland in mouth in which two types of enzymes are found, *ptyalin* and *maltase*. They convert starch into simple sugar and make it digestible.
⇨ In human secretion of saliva is approximately 1.5 litre per day.
⇨ The nature of saliva is acidic (pH 6.8).
⇨ From the mouth the food reach into stomach through food pipe.
⇨ No digestion takes place in food pipe.

Digestion in Stomach
⇨ The foods lies approximately for four hours in stomach.
⇨ After reaching the food in stomach gastric glands secretes the gastric juice. This is a light yellow acidic liquid.
⇨ Hydrochloric acid secreted from the Oxyntic cells of the stomach kills all the bacteria coming with food and accelerates the reaction of enzymes.
⇨ Hydrochloric acid makes the food acidic by which ptyalin reaction of the saliva end.
⇨ The enzymes in the gastric juice of stomach are – Pepsin and Renin.
⇨ Pepsin breaks down the protein into peptones.
⇨ Renin breaks down the Caseinogen into Casein.

Digestion in Duodenum

➪ As soon as the food reaches the duodenum bile juice from liver combines with it. Bile juice is an alkaline and it turns the acidic medium of food into alkaline.

➪ Here, pancreatic juice from pancreas combines with food. It contains three types of enzymes :

(i) Trypsin : It converts the protein and peptone into polypeptides and amino acid.

(ii) Amylase : It converts the starch into soluble sugar.

(iii) Lipase : It converts the emulsified fats into glycerol and fatty acids.

Small Intestine

➪ Here, the process of digestion completed and absorption of digested foods start.

➪ From the wall of small intestine, intestinal juices secretes. The following enzymes contain:

(i) *Erepsin* : It converts the remaining protein and peptone into amino acids.

(ii) *Maltase* : It converts the maltose into glucose.

(iii) *Sucrase* : It converts the sucrose into glucose and fructose.

(iv) *Lactase* : It converts the lactose into glucose and galactose.

(v) *Lipase* : It converts the emulsified fats into glycerol and fatty acids.

Intestinal juice is alkaline in nature.

In a healthy people approximately 2 litres of intestinal juice secretes everyday.

3. **Absorption :** Reaching of digested foods into blood is called absorption.

➪ The absorption of digested foods takes place through small intestinal villi.

4. **Assimilation :** Use of absorbed food in the body is called Assimilation.

5. **Defecation :** Undigested food reaches into large intestine where bacteria turns it into *faeces*, which is excreted through anus.

Summary of Digestion

	Gland Juice		Enzyme	Edible Substance	After Reaction
1.	Saliva	(i)	Ptylin	Starch	Maltose
		(ii)	Maltase	Maltose	Glucose
2.	Gastric juice	(i)	Pepsin	Protein	Peptones
		(ii)	Rennin	Casein	Calcium paracasein
3	Pancreatic juice	(i)	Trypsin	Protein	Polypeptides

		(ii)	Amylase	Starch	Sugar
		(iii)	Lipase	Fat	Fatty acid and glycerol
4.	Intestinal juice	(i)	Erepsin	Protein	Amino acid
		(ii)	Maltase	Maltose	Glucose
		(iii)	Lactase	Lactose	Glucose and fructose
		(iv)	Sucrase	Sucrose	Glucose and glactose
		(v)	Lipase	Fat	Fatty acid and glycerol

The main organs participating in digestion:

Liver: This is the largest gland of the human body. Its weight is approximately 1.5 – 2 kilogram.

⇨ Bile is secreted through liver only. This bile accelerate the reaction of enzymes present in the intestine.

⇨ Liver convert excess of amino acid into ammonia by deamination. These ammonia are further converted into urea by ornithine cycle. Urea comes out from body through kidney.

⇨ Liver converts some quantity of protein into glucose during deficiency of carbohydrate.

⇨ In carbohydrates metabolism liver converts the excess of glucose found in blood into glycogen and stores it into hepatic Cell as reserve nutrients. If the necessity of glucose arises the liver convert reserve glycogen into glucose. Thus, it regulates the quantity of glucose in the blood.

⇨ In case of decrease of fat in food liver converts some of the parts of the carbohydrates into fat.

⇨ The production of fibrinogen protein takes place by liver which helps in clotting of blood.

⇨ The production of Heparin protein takes place in liver which prohibit the clotting of blood inside the body.

⇨ The dead RBC is destroyed by the liver only.

⇨ The liver reserve some quantity of iron, copper and vitamin.

⇨ It helps in regulating the body temperature.

⇨ Liver is an important clue in investigating a person's death that has been due to poison in food.

Gall Bladder : Gall bladder is a pear shaped sac, in which the bile coming out of liver is stored.

⇨ Bile comes into the duodenum from gall bladder through the bile duct.

⇨ Secretion of bile into the duodenum takes place by reflex action.

⇨ Bile is a yellowish-green coloured alkaline liquid, whose pH value is 7.7.

⇨ The quantity of water is 85% and the quantity of bile pigment is 12% in water.

⇨ The Main functions of bile are as under :

(i) It makes the medium of food alkaline so that pancreatic juice can worked.

(ii) It kills the harmful bacteria coming with food.

(iii) It emulsifies the fats.

(iv) It accelerates the bowel movement of intestine by which digestive juices in the food mix well.

(v) It is helpful in the absorption of vitamin K and other vitamins mixed in fats.

In case of obstruction in bile duct, liver cells stop taking bilirubin from blood. As a result, bilirubin spreads throughout the body. This is called *jaundice*.

Pancreas : This is the second largest gland of the human body. It acts as simultaneously endocrine and exocrine type of gland.

➪ Pancreatic juice secretes out of it in which 9.8% water and the remaining parts contain salt and enzymes. It is alkaline liquid, whose pH value is 7.5 – 8.3. It contains the enzymes which can digest all the three types of food materials (like carbohydrates, fat and protein), therefore it is called complete digestive juice.

Islets of Langerhans : This is a part of the Pancreas.

➪ It was discovered by the medical scientist Langerhans.

➪ From its β cell- insulin, from α cell-glucagons and from δ cell-somatostaintin hormones are secreted :

Insulin : It is secreted by β-Cell of islets of Langerhans which is a part of the pancreas.

➪ It was discovered by Banting and Best in the year 1921.

➪ It controls the process of making glycogen from glucose.

➪ Diabetes is caused due to the deficiency of insulin.

➪ Excessive flow of insulin causes Hypoglycemia in which one loses the reproducing capacity and vision deterioration.

Glucagon : It re-converts the glycogen into glucose.

Somatostatin : This is a polypeptide hormone which increases the duration of assimilation of food.

(b) Circulatory System

The discovery of blood circulation was done by *William Harvey in* the year 1628.

There are four parts under it –

(i) Heart (ii) Arteries (iii) Veins and (iv) Blood.

Heart : It remains safe in the *pericardial membrane*. Its weight is approximately 300 grams.

Heart of the human is made up of four chambers. In the anterior side there is a *right auricle* and a *left auricle*. In the posterior side of the heart there is a *right ventricle* and a *left ventricle* persist.

➪ Between the right auricle and the right ventricle there is a *tricuspid valve*.

➪ Between the left auricle and left ventricle there is a *bicuspid valve*.

- The blood vessels carrying the blood from the body towards the heart is called *vein*.
- In the vein there is impure blood i.e. carbon dioxide mixed blood. Its exception is pulmonary vein, which always carry pure blood.
- Pulmonary vein carries the blood from lungs to left auricle. It has pure blood.
- The blood vessels carrying the blood from the heart towards the body is called *artery*.
- In artery there is pure blood i.e. oxygen mixed blood. Its exception is pulmonary artery.
- Pulmonary artery carries the blood from right ventricle to lungs. It contains impure blood.
- In the right part of the heart, there remains impure blood i.e. carbon dioxide mixed blood and in the left part of the heart there remains pure blood i.e. oxygen mixed blood.
- The artery carrying blood to the muscles of the heart are called *coronary arteries*. Any type of hindrance in it causes heart attack.

Course of circulation : Mammals have double circulation. It mean blood have to cross two times from heart before circulating throughout the body.

- Right auricle recieve impure blood from the body which goes into right ventricle. From here the blood went into pulmonary artery which send it to the lung for purification. After purification it is collected by pulmonary vein which bring it back to heart in left auricle. From auricle it went into left ventricle. Now this purified blood is went into aorta for different organ of body.

This circulation is done is a cardiac cycle.

- **Cardiac cycle:** Rhythmic systole (Contraction) and diastole (relaxation) of auricle and ventricle constitutes a cardiac cycle.
- **Heart beat:** Heart keeps beating rhythmically throughout the life. There is a node from which originate contraction of heart.
  (i) **Sino auricular node (SA node) :** It is a specialised area of cardiac muscle fiber in right auricle. SA node is also known as *pace maker* as it generates each wave of cardiac impulse.
  (ii) **Auriculo-Ventricular node (AV node) :** AV node is present close to the interatrial septum near the right AV aperture. Wave of contraction is picked up by AV node which spread through.
- Wave of excitation is picked up by AV node which spread through AV bundle of muscles fibers present on inter artrial septum as well as interventricular septum.
- **Artificial pace maker :** When SA node becomes defective or damaged, the cardiac impulses do not generate. This can be cured by surgical grafting of an artificial pace maker an electric device in the chest of the patient. It stimulate the heart electrically at regular intervals.

⇨ Systole and diastole of the heart are collectively called *heart beat*. In the normal condition the heart of the human beats 72 times and in a single beat it pumps approximately 70 ml blood.

⇨ The blood pressure of a normal human is 120/80. (Systolic – 120 and Diastolic – 80).

⇨ Blood pressure is measured by *sphygmomanometer*.

⇨ *Thyroxin* and *adrenaline* are the hormones which independently controls the heart beat.

⇨ The CO_2 present in the blood accelerates the heart beat by reducing the pH.

(c) Lymph Circulatory System

⇨ The light yellow fluid found in the inter-cellular intervals between different tissues and cells is called *lymph*.

⇨ Lymph is a fluid whose composition is like blood plasma, in which nutrient, oxygen and various other substances are present.

⇨ The corpuscles found in lymph are called *lymphocytes*. In fact, these are White Blood Corpuscles (WBC).

⇨ Lymph flows only in one direction from tissue towards heart.

Functions of lymph :

(i) The lymphocytes present in lymph helps to prevents the body from diseases by killing the harmful bacteria.

(ii) Lymph form the lymphocytes,

(iii) The node found in lymph vessels are called *lymph node* works as a filter in the human body.

(iv) Lymph helps in healing the wounds.

(v) Lymph circulates different material from tissues to veins.

(d) Excretory System

Excretion : Removal of nitrogenous substances formed during metabolism from the body of human is called *excretion*. Normally excretion means the release of nitrogenous excretory substances like urea, ammonia, uric acid etc.

The main excretory organs of human are as follows –

(i) Kidneys, (ii) Skin, (iii) Liver and (iv) Lungs.

(i) **Kidneys :** The main excretory organ in human and other mammals is a pair of kidneys. Its weight is 140 grams. There are two parts of it. Outer Part is called *cortex* and the inner part is called *medulla*. Each kidney is made up of approximately 1,30,00000 kidney ducts which are called *nephrons*. Nephron is the structural & functional unit of the kidney. There is a cup like structure in the every nephron called *Bowman's capsule*. Glomerulus of thin blood vessels are found in the Bowman's capsule which is made up of two types of arterioles.

(i) **Afferent arteriole :** Which carries the blood to the glomerulus.

(ii) **Efferent arteriole :** By which the blood is taken out of the glomerulus.

⇨ The process of filtration of liquids into the cavity of Bowman's capsule, is called *ultra filtration.*

⇨ The main function of the kidneys is purification of blood plasma i.e. to excrete the unwanted nitrogenous waste substances through urination.

⇨ The supply of blood to kidneys takes place in large quantity in comparison to other organs.

⇨ In the kidneys average 125 ml per minute blood is filtrated i.e. 180 liters per day. Out of it 1.45 liters urine is formed daily and the remaining is absorbed back by the cells of nephron and mix into the blood.

⇨ In the normal urine there is 95% water, 2% salt, 2.7% urea and 0.3% uric acid.

⇨ The colour of the urine is light yellow due to the presence of *urochromes* in it. Urochrome is formed by the dissotiation of haemoglobin.

⇨ Urine is acidic. Its pH value is 6.

⇨ The stone formed in the kidneys is made up of calcium oxalate.

(i) **Skin :** Oil gland and sweat glands found in the skin respectively secretes *sebum* and *sweat.*

(ii) **Liver:** Liver cells play the main role in excretion by converting more and more amino acids and ammonia of blood into urea.

(iii) **Lungs :** The lungs excretes two types of gaseous substances carbon dioxide and water vapour. The excretion of some substances like garlic, onion and some spices in which vapour component excreted by the lungs.

Different Animals and excretory parts

	Animal	Excretory parts
1.	Unicellular animal	By diffusion through general body surface
2.	Animals of Porifera Phylum	By general body surface contractile vocoule
3.	Coelenterates	Directly by cells.
4.	Flat worm	By flame cells.
5.	Animals of Annelida Phylum	By nephridia.
6.	Arthropods	By Malpighian tubules.
7.	Curstaceans	Antennal gland
8.	Mollusca	By urinary organ.
9.	Vertebrate	Mainly by kidneys

Hemodialysis : Process of removal of excess urea from the blood of patient using artificial kidney.

(e) Nervous System

Under this system thin thread like nerves are spread throughout the body. After receiving the information of environmental changes from the sensitive organs, it spreads them speedly like electrical impulses and establishes working and coordination among different organs.

Nervous system of human is divided into three parts :

(1) Central nervous system   (2) Peripheral nervous system

(3) Autonomic nervous system.

1. **Central Nervous System :** Part of the nervous system which keeps control on the whole body and on nervous system itself is called Central *Nervous System*. The Central Nervous System of human is made up of two parts – Brain and Spinal Cord.

Brain is covered by membrane called *meninges*. It is situated in a bony box called *craninum* which protect it from external injury.

I. Brain

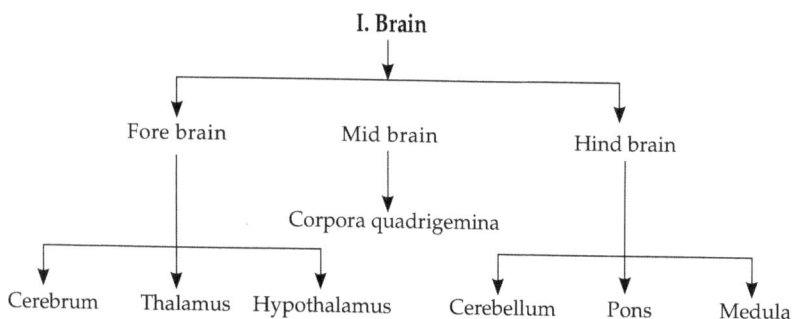

Fore brain   Mid brain   Hind brain

Corpora quadrigemina

Cerebrum   Thalamus   Hypothalamus   Cerebellum   Pons   Medula

(A) **Fore Brain :** The weight of the brain of the human is 1350 grams.

  (i) **The function of the Cerebrum :** This is the most developed part of the brain. This is the centre of wisdom, memory, will power, movements, knowledge and thinking. The analysis and coordination of muscular movement received from sense organs.

 (ii) **The function of thalamus :** It is the centre of the pain, cold and heat.

(iii) **The function of hypothalamus :** It controls the hormonal secretion from endocrine glands. Hormones secreted from posterior pituitary gland secrete through it. This is the centre of hunger, thirst, temperature control, love, hate etc. Blood pressure, metabolism of water, sweat, anger, joy etc. are controlled by it.

(B) The function of Corpora quadrigemina: This is the centre of control on vision and hearing power.

(C) Hind Brain

(i) Function of cerebellum : It is some what at the back of head and consist of two cerebellar hemisphere like cerebrum. It is large reflex centre for coordination of muscular body movements and maintenance of posture.

(ii) Pons : It act as bridge carrying ascending and descending tracts between brain and spinal cord.

(iii) Medulla : It is posterior most part of brain and continuous into the spinal cord. It connect and communicate the brain with spinal cord. It contains the cardiac respiratory and vasomotor centres that control complex activity like heart action, respiration, coughing, sneezing etc.

➪ The brain of the human is covered in the cranium which protects it from external injury. Brain is covered by membrane called *meanings*.

➪ **Spinal cord :** The posterior region of the medulla oblongata forms the spinal cord. Its main functions are :

(a) Coordination and control of reflex actions i.e. it works as the centre of the reflex actions.

(b) It carries the wave coming out of brain.

Note : *Reflex action was first discovered by the scientist, Marshall Hall.*

2. **Peripheral Nervous System :** Peripheral Nervous System is made up of the nerves arising from brain and spinal cord. These are called cranial and spinal nerves respectively. There are sensory, motor and mixed nerve.

➪ There are 12 pairs of cranial nerves and 31 pairs of spinal cord found in a human.

➪ The unit of nervous tissues is called *Neuron* or *nerve cell*.

3. **Autonomic Nervous System:** Autonomic Nervous System is made up of some brain nerves and some spinal cord nerves. It supplies nerves to all the internal organs and blood vessel of the body. *Langley*, first presented the concept of Autonomic Nervous System in the year 1921. There are two parts of Autonomic Nervous System:

(i) Sympathetic Nervous System

(ii) Parasympathetic Nervous System.

Functions of Sympathetic Nervous System :

(i) It narrows the blood vessels in the skin.

(ii) By its action hair gets erected.

(iii) It reduces the secretion of salivary glands.

(iv) It increases the heart beat.

(v) It increase the secretion of sweat glands.

(vi) It stretches the pupil of eye ball.

(vii) It relax the muscles of urinary bladder.

(viii) It reduces the speed of contraction & relaxation of intestine.

(ix) The rate of respiration increase.

(x) It increases the blood pressure.

(xi) It increases the sugar level in the blood.

(xii) It increases the number of Red Blood Corpuscles in the blood.

(xiii) It helps in clotting of blood.

(xiv) Collective impact of this affects fear, pain and anger.

Functions of Parasympathetic Nervous System :

The functions of this system is normally the opposite of Sympathetic Nervous System. For example :

(i) It widens the lumen of blood vessels but except the coronary blood vessels.

(ii) It increases the secretion of saliva and other digestive juices.

(iii) The contraction of pupil is caused by this.

(iv) It creates contraction in the other muscles of the urinary bladder.

(v) It creates contraction and motion in intestinal walls.

(vi) The effect of this nervous system collectively creates the occasion of rest and joy.

(f) Skeletal System

The skeletal system of human is made up of two parts :

(a) Axial skeleton and

(b) Appendicular skeleton.

(a) **Axial skeleton :** The skeleton, which makes the main axis of the body is called *axial skeleton*. Skull, vertebral column and bones of chest comes under it. There are 80 bones in axial skeleton.

(i) **Skull:** There are 29 bones in it. Out of these, 8 bones jointly protect the brain of the human. The structure made up of these bones is called *forehead*. All the bones of the fore head remain joined strongly by the sutures. There are 14 bones in addition to this which form the face. Six ear ossicles and one hyoid bone.

(ii) **Vertebral Column :** The vertebral column of the human is made up of 33 vertebra. All the vertebra are joined by intervertebral disc. Vertebra is made flexible by these intervertebral disc. We divide the whole vertebral column into the following parts :

1.	Cervical region	7 vertebras
2.	Thoracic region	12 vertebras
3.	Lumber region	5 vertebras
4.	Sacral region	(1) 5 vertebras
5.	Caudal region	(1) 4 vertebras
		Total – 33

➩ Its first vertebra which is called *atlas vertebra* holds the skull.

Functions of vertebral column :

(i) Holds the head.

(ii) It provides the base to the neck and body.

(iii) It helps the human in standing, walking etc.

(iv) It provides flexibility to the neck and body by which a human can move its neck and body in any direction.

(v) It provides protection to spinal cord.

     (b) Appendicular skeleton : The following are the parts of it -

        (i) Foot bones – Both hands and feet have 118 bones.

        (ii) To hold the fore limb and hind limb on the axial skeleton in human there are two girdles.

➩ The girdle of fore limb is called *pectoral girdle* and girdle of hind limb is called *pelvic girdle.*

➩ Pectoral girdle joined with forelimb is called *humerus* and the bone from pelvic girdle join to hindlimb is called *femur.*

Functions of the skeletal system :

(i) To provide a definite shape to the body.

(ii) To provide protection to soft parts of the body.

(iii) To provide a base to the muscles for joining.

(iv) To help in respiration and nutrition.

(v) To form Red Blood Corpuscles.

➩ The total number of bones in a human's body   –   206

➩ The total number of bones during childhood   –   300

➩ The total number of bones of head   –   29
(fore head-8, facial-14, ear-6, hyoid -1)

➩ The total number of bones in vertebral column, initially–33
After development   – 26 (5 sacral fuse into 1 and 4 caudal fuse into 1)

➩ The total number of bones of ribs   24

➩ The largest bone of the body   *Femur* (bone of thigh)

➩ The smallest bone of the body   *Stapes* (bone of ear)

The name and number of bones of some specific regions :

Ear bones	Maleus	(2)	Upper arm	Humerus	(2)
	Incus	(2)	Fore arm	Radio ulna	(2)
	Stapes	(2)	Wrist	Carpals	(16)
Palm	Meta carpals	(10)	Fingers	Phalanges	(28)
Thigh	Femur	(2)	Hind limb	Tibia-fibula	(4)
Knee	Patella	(2)	Ankle	Tarsal	(14)
Sole	Meta tarsal	(10)			

Note : *(i) The muscles and bones are join together by tendon.*
(ii) The muscle which join bone to bone is called ligaments.

(g) Endocrine System

(a) **Exocrine glands :** Gland which have duct are called *exocrine gland*. Secretion of enzymes pass through it. Example - *Lactic gland, Sweat gland, Mucous gland, Salivary gland etc.*

(b) **Endocrine gland :** These are *ductless gland*. Hormones are secreted by these gland. Hormones are sent to the different parts of the body through blood plasma. Example - *Pituitary gland, Thyroid gland, Parathyroid gland etc.*

Functions and effect of the main endocrine system of the human body and hormone secreted by them –

1. **Pituitary gland :** It is situated in a depression of the sphenoid bone of the fore head. This is called *sella – tunica.*

⇨ Its weight is approximately 0.6 grams.

⇨ This is also known as master gland. Pirutary gland is controlled by hypothalenus.

The functions of the hormones secreted by Pituitary gland :

(i) **STH hormone (Somatotropic hormone) :** It controls the growth of the body especially the growth of bones. By the excessiveness of STH *gigantism* and *acromegaly* are caused, in which height of the human grows abnormally. Lack of STH causes *dwarfism* in human.

(ii) **TSH hormone (Thyroid Stimulating Hormone) :** It stimulates the thyroid gland to secrete hormone.

(iii) **ACTH Hormone (Adrenocorticotropic Hormone) :** It controls the secretion of adrenal cortex.

(iv) **GTH Hormone (Growth Hormone) :** It controls the functions of gonads. This is of two types :

(a) **FSH Hormone (Follicle – Stimulating Hormone) :** In male it stimulates spermatogenesis in the seminiferous tubules of the testis. In female, it stimulates the Graffian follicles of the ovary to secret the hormone *Oestrogen.*

(b) **LH Hormone (Luteiniging Hormone)** : Interstitial cell stimu-lating hormone — secretion of *testosterone* hormone takes place in male and in case of female *estrogen* hormone secreted.

(v) **LTH Hormone (Lactogenic Hormone)** : Its main function is to stimulate secretion of milk in breasts for infants.

(vi) **ADH Hormone (Antidiuretic Hormone):** It causes increase in blood pressure. It is helpful in maintaining the water balance in the body and reduce the volume of urine.

2.   **Thyroid gland** : This is situated below the larynx on both side of respiratory trachea in throat of human.

⇨   The hormones secreted by it are Thyroxine and Triodothyronine. Iodine is secretes in more quantity.

Functions of Thyroxin :

(i) It increases the speed of cellular respiration.

(ii) It is necessary for the normal growth of the body particularly for the development of bones, hair etc.

(iii) The normal functions of reproductive organs depend on the activeness of thyroid gland.

(iv) It controls the water balance of the body in coordination with the hormones of pituitary gland.

Diseases Caused by the Deficiency of Thyroxin :

(i)   **Cretinism:** This disease affects the children. The mental and physical retardness of the child.

(ii) **Myxedema:** In this disease which normally attack during youth the metabolism does not take place properly which causes reduction in heart beat and blood pressure.

(iii) **Hypothyroidism :** This disease is caused due to a chronic deficiency of thyroxin hormone. Due to this diseases the normal reproduction is not possible. Sometimes due to this disease human becomes dumb and deaf.

(iv) **Goitre :** This disease is caused by the deficiency of iodine in food. In this disease the shape of the thyroid gland enlarges abnormally.

Diseases caused by the Excessiveness of Thyroxin :

Exopthalmic Goitre : In this disease eyes get bulging out of the eye socket with increased metabolic rate.

3.   **Parathyroid gland :** This is situated in the right back of the thyroid gland of the throat. Two hormones are secreted by it:

(i)   **Parathyroid hormone :** This hormone is secreted when there is a deficiency of calcium in the blood.

(ii) **Calcitonin:** This hormone is released when there is excess of calcium in the blood is present.

Hence, hormone secreted by parathyroid gland controls the quantity of calcium in blood.

4. **Adrenal gland :** There are two parts of this gland - (i) outer part is cortex and (ii) inner part is medulla.

Hormones secreted by cortex and their function :

(i) **Glucocorticoids :** This controls the metabolism of carbohydrate, protein and fat.

(ii) **Mineralocorticoids :** Its main function is reabsorption of ion by kidney ducts and to control the quantity of other on in the body.

(iii) **Sex hormone:** It controls the sexual behaviour and secondary sexual characters.

Note : *(i) Cortex is essential for life. If this is extracted completely from the body, human will remain alive only for a week or two.*

(ii) In case of deformation of cortex, the process of metabolism gets disturbed; this disease is called Addison's disease.

Hormones secreted by Medulla and their function :

(i) *Epinephrine* – This is an amino acid.

(ii) *Nor epinephrine* – This is also an amino acid.

➪ The work of both the hormones is similar. These equally increase the relaxation and contraction of heart muscles. As a result, blood pressure increases and

➪ In case of sudden stop of heart beat, epinephrine is helpful in re-starting the heart beat.

➪ The hormone secreted by Adrenal gland is called fight flight, fright fight hormone.

5. **Gonads:**

(1) **Ovary :** The following hormones are secreted by this :

(i) **Estrogen :** It completes the increase of oviduct.

(ii) **Progesterone :** It stimulates the thickening of uterus lining during ovarien cycle.

(iii) **Relaxin:** During pregnancy it is found in uterus and placenta. This hormone smoothens the pubic symphysix and it widens the uterine cervix so that a child is delivered easily.

(2) **Testes:** The hormone secreted by it is called testosterone. It motivates the sexual behaviour and growth of secondary sexual characters.

(h) Respiratory System

➪ The most important organ of the respiratory system of human is lungs where the exchange of gases takes place.

➪ All those organs comes under respiratory system which help in exchange of gases are – Nasal passage, Pharynx, Larynx or Voice box, Trachea, Bronchi, Bronchioles, Lungs etc.

- **Nasal passage :** Its main function is related to sniffing. Its inner cavity is lined with mucous membrane. This secretes approximately ½ litre of mucous everyday. This prevents the particles of sand, bacteria or other small organisms from entering into the body. It makes the air wet entering into the body and equalises it with the temperature of the body.
- **Pharynx :** It is situated behind the nasal cavity.
- **Larynx or Voice box:** The part of the respiratory way which connects the pharynx with trachea is called *Larynx or voice box*. Its main function is to produce sound. At the larynx entrance gate there is a thin blade-like door, which is called *epiglottis*. When any food particle is swallowed it closes the glottis, as a result food does not enter into respiration pipe.
- **Trachea :** It enters into the thoracic cavity. The two main branches of trachea are called *bronchi*. Right bronchi enters into the right lungs after being divided into three branches. Left bronchi enters into the left lungs after being divided into only two branches.
- **Lungs:** There is a pair of lungs in the thoracic cavity. Its colour is red and looks like sponge. Right lung is larger in comparison to left lung. Each lung is surrounded by a membrane which is called *pleural membrane*. There is a network of blood capillaries . Here Oxygen enters into the blood and CO_2 comes out.

The process of respiration can be divided into four parts :

1. External respiration.   2. Transportation of gases.
3. Internal respiration.   4. Cellular respiration.

1. **External respiration :** This is divided into two parts –
   (a) Breathing   (b) Exchange of gases.
   (a) **Breathing :** In lungs air is taken and given out at a certain rate which is called *breathing*.

Mechanism of Breathing :

(i) **Inspiration :** At this stage, air from the environment enters into the lungs through the nasal passage, due to increases in the dimension of thoracic cavity a low pressure is formed in the lungs and air enters into the lungs from environment. This air continues to enter until the pressure of air inside and outside the body became equal.

(ii) **Expiration :** In this process air comes out of the lungs. Constitution of air in Breathing

	Nitrogen	Oxygen	Carbon dioxide
The air inhaled	79%	21%	0.03%
The air exhaled	79%	17%	4%

Everyday approximately 400 ml water is excreted through breathing.

(b) **Exchange of gases** : The exchange of gases takes place inside the lungs. This gaseous exchange takes place on the basis of concentration gradient through normal diffusion.

The exchange of oxygen and carbon dioxide gases takes place due to their difference in partial pressures. The direction of diffusion of both.

2. **Transportation of gases** : The process of reaching of gases (oxygen and carbon dioxide) from lungs to the cells of body and coming back again to the lungs is called the transportation of gases.

➪ Transportation of oxygen takes place by haemoglobin present in blood.

➪ Transportation of carbon dioxide from cells to lung takes place by haemoglobin only to the extent of 10 to 20%.

➪ Transportation of carbon dioxide takes place through circulation of blood :

(i) **By mixing with plasma** : Carbon dioxide forms carbonic acid after mixing in plasma. Transportation of 7% carbon dioxide takes place in this form.

(ii) **In the form of bicarbonates** : 70% part of carbon dioxide in the form of bicarbonates is transported. It mixes with potassium and sodium of blood and forms potassium bicarbonate and sodium bicarbonate.

3. **Internal respiration:** Inside the body, gaseous exchange takes place between blood and tissue fluid which is called *internal respiration.*

Note : *The gaseous exchange in lungs is called external respiration.*

4. **Cellular respiration** : Glucose is oxidised by oxygen reached into the cell. This process is called *cellular respiration.*

Types of cellular respiration :

Respiration is of two type

(a) **Anaerobic respiration** : If the oxidation of food takes place in absence of oxygen. During this only 2 ATP molecules are produced from one molecule of glucose. Final product of anaerobic respiration in animal tissue like skeletal muscle cell is lactic acid.

In yeast and certain bacteria ethyl alcohol or ethanol is produced.

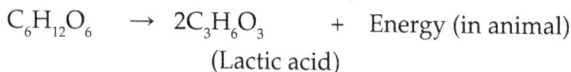

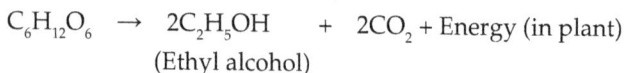

$$C_6H_{12}O_6 \quad \rightarrow \quad 2C_3H_6O_3 \quad + \quad \text{Energy (in animal)}$$
$$\text{(Lactic acid)}$$

$$C_6H_{12}O_6 \quad \rightarrow \quad 2C_2H_5OH \quad + \quad 2CO_2 + \text{Energy (in plant)}$$
$$\text{(Ethyl alcohol)}$$

(b) **Aerobic respiration** : It takes place in the presence of oxygen. The complete oxidation of glucose takes place. As a result CO_2 and H_2O is formed and energy is released in huge amount.

$C_6H_{12}O_6 + 6O_2 \rightarrow 6CO_2 + 6H_2O + 2870$ KJ energy. (38 ATP)

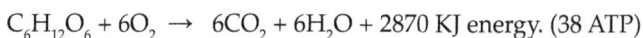

The complex process in cellular respiration is divided into two parts-

(i) Glycolysis (cytoplasm) (ii) Kreb's cycle (Mitochondria)

(i) **Glycolysis :** Its study was first done by *Embden Meyorh pathway*. Therefore, it is also called *EMP path*

⇨ Glycolysis is present in both types of respiration, Aerobic and Anaerobic. This process takes place in cytoplasm.

⇨ As a result of decomposition of one glucose atom in glycolysis two atoms of pyruvic acid is formed.

⇨ To start this process 2 atoms of ATP (Adenosine Triphosphate) takes part but at the end of the process 4 atoms ATP are obtained. Therefore, as a result of glycolysis 2 atom ATP are obtained i.e. 16000 calorie (2 × 8000) energy is obtained.

⇨ There is no need of oxygen in glycolysis. Hence, this process is similar in anaerobic respiration and aerobic respiration.

⇨ In this, four molecules of hydrogen formed which is used in converting NAD to $2NADH_2$.

(ii) Kreb's Cycle : It was described by *Hens Krebs* in 1937.

⇨ This is also called *Citric Acid Cycle or Tricarboxylic Cycle*.

⇨ This process is completed inside the Mitochondria in the presence of specific enzymes.

⇨ Two atoms of each ADP and ATP are formed.

⇨ In this cycle 4 pair of hydrogen atom are released.

⇨ The complete cycle is of 2 atom pyruvic acid, produce total 4 atoms of carbon dioxide.

⇨ In our system maximum ATP atoms are formed during Kreb's Cycle.

Production of energy : By the oxidation of pyruvic acid one atom of ATP, five atoms of NADH and one atom of $NADH_2$ are formed. From one atom of NADH three atoms of ATP and from one atom of $NADH_2$ two atoms of ATP are obtained. Hence, from one atom of pyruvic acid $1 + (3 \times 5) + (2 \times 1) = 18$ atoms of ATP are formed. From one atom of glucose two atoms of pyruvic acid are formed, by which 36 atoms of ATP are released. During the glycolysis, two atoms of ATP are obtained. Hence, during respiration of one atom of glucose total $2 + 36 = 38$ ATP atoms are obtained.

Respiratory substances : Carbohydrate, fat and protein are the main respiratory substances. At first, oxidation of glucose takes place, then fat. After the consumption of carbohydrate and fat oxidation of protein start.

Note : *Respiration is a Catabolic Process. It also reduces the weight of the body.*

5. Nutrients

To maintain life organisms performs some basic function is called *nutrition*. Nutrition is one of the basic function of life in which intake of food, digestion, absorption, assimilation and egestion of undigested foods are included.

Nutrient: Nutrient are the substance by which an organism get energy or it is used for biosynthesis of its body.

For example carbohydrate and fat are the source of energy. Whereas proteins and minerals are the nutrient used for biosynthesis.

Carbohydrate : Carbohydrates are organic compounds in which the ratio of Carbon, Hydrogen and Oxygen is 1 : 2 : 1. Carbohydrate in the form of sugar and starch are major intake in animals and human. 50 to 75% energy is obtained by oxidation of carbohydrate. Carbohydrate containing aldehyde group is called *aldose* and with ketone group is called *ketose*. Carbohydrates are derivatives of polyhydroxy alcohols.

Classification of carbohydrate : Carbohydrates are classified into three Major group.

(a) **Monosaccharides :** These are the simple sugar made up of single polyhydroxy or ketone unit. Most abundant monosaccharides found in nature is glucose containing six carbon atom. Triose, tetrose, pentoses, heptoses are the type of monosaccharides.

(b **Oligosaccharides :** When 2 to 10 monosaccharides join together they form oligosaccharides. They are usually crystalline in nature and sweet in test. Maltose, sucrose, lactose are disaccharides made up of two monosaccharides.

(c) **Polysaccharides:** These are the compound of sugar which are formed due to joining large number of monosaccharide. There are insoluble and tasteless. Some example of polysaccharides are *starch, glycogen, cellulose, chitin* etc.

Function of Carbohydrate

1. Carbohydrate works as fuel. During the process of respiration, glucose break into CO_2 & H_2O with the release of energy. One gram of glucose gives 4.2 kilo calories energy.
2. Nucleic acids are polymers of nucleosides and nucleotides and contain pentose sugar.
3. Lactose of milk is formed from glucose and glactose.
4. Glucose is used for the formation of fat and amino acid.
5. Carbon skeleton of monosaccharides is used in the formation of fatty acid, chitin, cellulose etc.

Source of Carbohydrate : Wheat, rice, maize, sweet potato, potato and other plant and animals are the sources of carbohydrate.

2. Protein: Protein word was first used by *J. Berzelius*. This is a complex organic compound made up of 20 type of amino acids. Approximately 15% of the human body is made up of protein. Nitrogen is present in protein in addition to C, H & O.

Twenty two types of protein is necessary for human body, out of which 12 are synthesized by body itself and remaining 10 are obtained by food are called essential amino acid.

Types of Proteins :

On the basis of chemical composition

It is divided into three types.

(1) Simple Protein : It consists of only amino acid.

Example— *Albumins, Globulins, Histories* etc.

(2) Conjugated Protein : Having some another chemical compounds in addition to amino acid.

Example : *Chromoprotein, Glycoprotein* etc.

(3) Derived Protein : It is derived from the partial digestion of natural proteins or its hydrolysis.

Example— *Peptone, Peptide, Proteinase* etc.

Functions of Protein :

(i) It takes part in the formation of cells, protoplasm and tissues.

(ii) These are important for physical growth. Physical growth hampers by its deficiency. Lack of proteins causes *Kwashiorkor* and *Marasmus* diseases in children.

(iii) In case of necessity these provide energy to the body.

(iv) These control the development of genetic characters.

(v) These are helpful in conduction also.

Kwashiorkor : In this disease hands and legs of children get slimmed and the stomach comes out.

Marasmus : In this disease muscles of children are loosened.

3. Fats : Fat is an ester of glycerol and fatty acid.

In these carbon, hydrogen and oxygen are present in different quantities, but proportionally less oxygen than carbohydrate.

Normally *fat* remains as solid at 20°C temperature, but if it is in liquid form at this temperature, this is called *oil*.

Fatty acids are of two types – Saturated and unsaturated. Unsaturated faty acids are found in fish oil and vegetable oil. Only coconut oil and palm oil are the examples of saturated oil.

9.3 kilo calorie energy is liberated from 1 gram fat.

Normally an adult person should get 20-30% of energy from fat.

Main functions of fat:

(i) It provides energy to the body.

(ii) It remains under the skin and prevents the loss of heat from the body.

(iii) It make the food material testy.

(iv) It protects different parts of the body from Injury.

Due to the lack of fat skin gets dried, weight of the body decreases and the development of the body checked.

Due to the excessiveness of fat the body gets fatty, heart disease takes place and blood pressure increases.

4. Vitamins : Vitamin was invented by *Sir F. G. Hopkins.* The term vitamin was coined by *Funk.*

Vitamins are organic compound required in minute quantities. No calorie is obtained from it, but it is very important in regulating chemical reactions in metabolism of the body.

On the basis of solubility, vitamins are of two types :

(i) *Vitamin soluble in water* : Vitamin-B and Vitamin-C.

(ii) *Vitamin soluble in fat* : Vitamin-A, Vitamin-D, Vitamin-E and Vitamin-K.

The diseases caused by the deficiency of vitamins and their sources

Vitamin	Chemical name	Deficiency diseases	Sources
Vitamin-A	Retinol	Colour blindness, Xerophthalmia	Milk, Egg, Cheese, Green vegetable fish liver oil
Vitamin-B_1	Thymine	Beriberi	Ground nut, Rapseed, Dried Chilli, Pulses, Liver, Egg, Vegetables etc.
Vitamin-B_2	Riboflavin	Cracking of skin, red-dish eye, cracking of tongue	Meat, Green vegetables, Milk etc.
Vitamin-B_3	Pantothenic acid	Whitening of hair, mentally retardness	Meat, Milk, Nut, Tomato, Sugarcane etc.
Vitamin-B_5	Nicotinamide or Niacin	Pellagra or 4-D Syndrome	Meat, Ground nut, Potato, Tomato, Leafy vegetables etc.
Vitamin-B_6	Pyridoxine	Anaemia, skin disease	Liver, Meat, Grains etc.

Vitamin-B$_7$	Biotin	Paralysis, body pain, hair falling	Meat, Egg, Liver, Milk etc.
Vitamin-B$_{12}$	Cynocobalamin	Anaemia, jaundice Teroile Glutemic	Meat, Milk etc.
Folic acid	—	Anaemia, diarrhoea	Pulses, Liver, Vegetables, Eggs etc.
Vitamin-C	Ascorbic acid	Scurvy, Swelling of gums	Lemon, Orange, Tomato, Sour substances, Chilly, Sprouted grain etc.
Vitamin-D	Calciferol	Rickets (in children), Osteomalasia (in adults)	Fish liver oil, Milk, Eggs etc.
Vitamin-E	Tocopherol	Less fertility	Leafy vegetables, Milk, Butter, Sprouted wheat, Vegetable oil etc.
Vitamin-K	Phylloquinone	Non-clotting of blood	Tomato, Soybean oil Green vegetables, etc.

⇨ Cobalt is found in Vitamin-B$_{12}$

⇨ Synthesis of vitamins cannot be done by the cells and it is fulfilled by the vitamin foods.

⇨ However, synthesis of Vitamin-D and K takes place in our body. Synthesis of Vitamin-D takes place by the ultra violet rays present in the sunlight through cholesterol (Irgesterol) of skin.

⇨ Vitamin-K is synthesized in our colon by the bacteria and from there it is absorbed.

6. **Minerals :** Mineral is a homogenous inorganic material needed for body. These control the metabolism of body.

Important Minerals and Their Functions

Minerals	Daily quantity	Main sources	Functions
Sodium (as sodium chloride)	2 – 5 gram	Normal salt, fish, meat, eggs, milk etc.	It normally found in external fluid of cell and is related to following functions: Contractions of muscles, In the transmission of nerve impulses in nerve fiber. Control of positive electrolyte balance in body etc.

Potassium	1 gram	Approximately all edibles	It is normally found in protoplasm. It is important for following different chemical reactions in cells: Muscular contraction, nerve conduction, maintenance of positive electrolyte in body etc.
Calcium	Approx. 1.2 gram	Milk, cheese, eggs, grains, gram, fish etc.	This provides strength to bones and teeth with vitamin, Important role in blood formation, Related with muscular contruction. Help in clotting the blood etc.
Phosphorus	1.2 gram	Milk, cheese, Bajra, green leaf vegetables, etc.	This provides strength to bones and teeth, in coordination with calcium.
Iron	25 mg (boy) 35 mg (girl)	Albumen of egg, bread, Bajra, Banana, Spanich apple	Iron is important in formation of Red Blood Corpuscles and haemoglobin. This is important for tissue oxidation.
Iodine	20 mg	Sea fish, sea food, green leaf vegetables, Iodized salt.	This is important for synthesis of thyroxin hormone secreted by Thyroid gland.
Magnesium	Very small quantity	Vegetables	For functioning of muscular system and nervous system.
Zinc	Very small quantity	Liver and fishes	For insulin functioning.
Copper	Very small quantity	Meat, fish, liver and grains.	Formation of haemoglobin and bones and as a conductor of electron.
Cobalt	Very small quantity	Meat, fish and water	For synthesis of RBC and Vitamin B_{12}

7. Water: Human gets it by drinking. Water is the important component of our body. 65-75% weight of the body is water.

Main functions of water :

1. Water controls the temperature of our body by sweating and vaporizing.
2. It is the important way of excretion of the excretory substances from the body.
3. Maximum organic chemical reactions in the body perform through hydrolysis.

Balance Diet: That nutrition, in which all the important nutrients for organism are available in sufficient quantity, is called *Balance Diet*.

Balance nutrition is obtained from Balance Diet, which is given in the chart below:

Edibles	Adult male			Adult female			Children		Boy	Girl
	N	M	Hard	N	M	Hard	1-3 yrs.	4-6 yrs.	10-18 yrs.	10-16 yrs.
Grain (wheat, rice)	400 g	520 g	670 g	410 g	440 g	575 g	175 g	270 g	420 g	380 g
Pulses	40 g	50 g	60 g	40 g	45 g	50 g	35 g	35 g	45 g	45 g
Leafy vegetables	40 g	40 g	40 g	100 g	100 g	50 g	40 g	50 g	50 g	50 g
Vegetables (other)	60 g	70 g	80 g	40 g	40 g	100 g	20 g	30 g	50 g	50 g
Milk	150 g	200 g	250 g	100 g	150 g	200 g	300 g	250 g	250 g	250 g
Tuber root	50 g	60 g	80 g	50 g	50 g	60 g	10 g	20 g	30 g	30 g
Sugar	30 g	35 g	55 g	20 g	20 g	40 g	30 g	40 g	45 g	45 g
Fat and oil	40 g	45 g	65 g	20 g	25 g	40 g	15 g	25 g	40 g	35 g

Necessary calorie for a human being :

	Nature of work	Male	Female
1.	Light worker	2000 calorie	2100 calorie
2.	Eight hours worker	3000 calorie	2500 calorie
3.	Hard worker	3600 calorie	3000 calorie

6. Human Diseases

Diseases caused by Protozoa :

	Disease	Affected organ	Parasites	Carrier	Symptoms
1.	Malaria	RBC & Liver	*Plasmodium*	Female Anophelies	Fever with shivering

2.	Pyorrhoea	Gums	*Entamoeba gingivelis*	—	Bleeding from gums.
3.	Sleeping sickness	Brain	*Trypanosoma*	Tse–Tse flies	Fever with severe sleep.
4.	Diarrhoea	Intestine	*Entamoeba histolytica*	—	Mucous & Diarrohea with blood.
5.	Kala-ajar	Bone marrow	*Leismania donovani*	Sand flies	High fever.

Charles Leveran discovered the Malaria Parasite, *plasmodium* in the blood of the affected person in the year 1880.

Ronald Ross (1897) confirmed the Malaria is caused by malaria parasite and told that mosquito is the carrier of it.

Diseases caused by Bacteria :

Disease	Affected organ	Name of Bacteria	Symptoms
Tetanus	Nervous system	*Clostridium Tetani*	High fever, spasm in body, Closing of jaws etc.
Cholera	Intestine	*Vibrio cholerae*	Continuous stool and vomiting.
Typhoid	Intestine	*Salmonella typhosa*	High fever, headache.
Tuberculosis	Lungs	*Mycobacterium tuberculosis*	Repeated coughing.
Diphtheria	Respiratory tube	*Corynebacterium diphtheriae*	Difficulty in respiration and suffocation.
Plague	Lungs, area between the two legs	*Pasteurella pesties*	Very high fever, muscular eruptions on the body.
Whooping cough	Respiratory system	*Hemophilis pertusis*	Continuous coughing
Pneumonia	Lungs	*Diplococcus pneumoniae*	High fever, swelling in lungs.
Leprosy	Nervous System Skin	*Mycobacterium leprae*	Spots on body, nerves affected.
Gonorrhea	Urinary Path	*Neisseria Gonorrhoeae*	Swelling in urinary path.
Syphilis	Urinary path	*Treponema pallidum*	Wounds in urinogenial tract

Note : *In the year 1882, German scientist Robert Koch discovered the bacteria of Cholera and T.B.*

Louis Pasteur discovered the vaccine of Rabies and pasteurization of milk.

Diseases caused by Viruses

	Disease	Affected organ	Name of virus	Symptoms
1.	AIDS	Defensive system (WBC)	HIV	Immune system of body became weak.
2.	Dengue fever	Whole body particularly head, eyes and joints.	Billions of virus	Pain in eyes, muscles, head and joints
3.	Polio	Throat, backbone Nerve.	Pilio virus	Fever, body pain, backbone and intestine cells are destroyed.
4.	Influenza (flu)	Whole body	Mixo virus	Suffocation, sneezing, restlessness.
5.	Chicken pox	Whole body	Variola virus	High fever, redish eruption on body.
6.	Small pox	Whole body	Varicella virus	Light fever, eruption of bile on body.
7.	Goitre	Parathyroid gland	—	Difficulty in opening the mouth with fever.
8.	Measles	Whole body	Morbeli virus	Redish eruptions on body
9.	Trachoma	Eyes	—	Reddish eyes, pain in eyes.
10.	Hepatitis or Jaundice	Liver	—	Yellow urine, Eyes and skin become yellow.
11.	Rabies	Nervous system	Rabies virus	The patient becomes mad with sever headache & high fever.

| 12. | Meningitis | Brain | — | High fever. |
| 13. | Herpes | Skin | Herpes | Swelling in skin. |

Note : *AIDS - Acquired Immuno Deficiency Syndrome.*

Elisa Test: *Test of HIV Virus (AIDS)*

Diseases caused by Protozoa :

(i) **Diarrhoea :** The reason of this disease is the presence of internal protozoa namely *Entamoeba histolytica* which is spread through house flies. It causes wounds in the intestine. Protein digesting enzyme, trypsin is destroyed in this. This disease is mostly found in children. Disease caused by helminthes.

(ii) **Filaria :** This disease is caused by *Wuchereia baoncrofti*. This worm is circulated by the stings of culex mosquitoes. This disease causes swelling in legs, testes and other parts of the body. This disease is also known as *Elephantiasis*.

Diseases caused by Fungus

(i) **Asthma :** The spores of the fungi, namely *Aspergillus fumigatus* reaches the lungs of the human and constitutes a net like formation, thus, obstructs the function of lungs. This is a infections disease.

(ii) **Athlete's foot :** This disease is caused by the fungi namely *Tenia Pedes*. This is a infections disease of skin which spreads mainly due to the cracking of feet.

(iii) **Scabies :** This disease is caused by the fungi namely *Acarus scabies*. In this disease the skin itches and white spots found on the skin.

(iv) **Baldness :** This is caused by the fungi namely *Taenia capitis*. Due to this hair of the head falls.

(v) **Ringworm :** This disease spreads through the fungi namely *Trycophyton Lerucosum*. This is a infections disease. Round red spot found on the skin.

Some Other Diseases

1. **Paralysis or Hemiplegia :** In this disease within a few minutes half of the body is paralyzed. The nerves of the paralyzed part become inactive.

   The reason of this disease is due to high blood pressure bursting of any nerve of brain or insufficient supply of blood to brain.

2. **Allergy :** Some substance like sand, smoke, chemical, clothes, cold are dangerous to some persons and there are reactions in their body, which causes various diseases. Itching, pimples, swelling in body, black spot, eczema etc. are the examples of allergy.

3. **Schizophrenia :** This is a mental disease which usually found in youth. The patient considers the imagination as a truth, not to the facts. These patients are lazy, emotionless etc. Electropathy is helpful in this disease.

4. **Epilepsy :** This disease is caused by the internal disturbance of brain. In this disease, foam coming out of the mouth and the patient falls down unconscious.

5. **Diplopia :** This disease is caused by the paralysis of muscles of the eyes, in which double image is formed.

6. **Bronchitis :** It is caused by the inflammation of tubes leading from the wind pipe to lungs.

7. **Colds :** This is highly infections disease and is caused by a virus which result in bad throat, headache and watery nose.

8. **Colic :** Severe pain in the abdomen caused by spasm of the internal organs usually the intestines.

9. **Delirium :** It is a serious mental disturbance occuring under the influence of poisonous drugs.

10. **Hydrophobia :** A disease cause by bite of a mad dog.

11. **Hyper metropia (long sightedness) :** One can see the object of longer distance but not the object of nearer one. It can be corrected by convex lens.

12. **Myopia (short sightedness):** In this disease person can see the object of nearer distance but can not see the object of longer distance. It is corrected by using concave lens.

13. **Leukaemia :** There is a great increase in the number of white blood corpuscles in system. Swelling of spleen takes place. Death occur within few days.

14. **Migrain :** An allergic disease in which there is a periodic attack of headache takes place. It is an incureble disease.

15. **Obesity :** Excessive fatness is called *obesity*.

16. **Piles :** There are a various vein in the rectum. Due to extra pressure on vein it prevent the free flow of blood creating problem. It is caused due to constipation.

17. **Rheumatism :** The symptiom of this disease is fever with joints Pain.

Other Disease

Atherosclerosis : Deposition of cholesterol particles in the lumen of arteries which prevent the flow of blood is called atherosclerosis.

Arteriosclerosis : Due to deposition of cholesterol and calcium salt arteries became stiff and rigid. It loses the property of elasticity due to which wall of arteries may rap fun.

Uremia : Presence of excess of urea in blood is called uremia, This is caused by malfunctioning of kidney.

Glgcosuria : Presence of excess of glucose urine is known as glycosuria.

Arthritis : It is disease in which inflammation of joints takes place.

Osteoporosis : It is a age dependent disorder of bone in which low bone mass and increased fragility takes place.

Hyperglycemia : It is disorder in which the concentration of glucose in the blood is high.

Hypoglycemia : It is a condition in which the concentration of glucose in the blood is very low.

Pneumonia : Acute inflamation of alveoli of lung.

Emphysema : It is the abnormal distension of alveoli which result in the loss of elasticity. Cigarette smoke and chronic bronchitis are two main causes.

Miscellaneous

1. Medicinal Discoveries

Inventions/Discoveries	Inventor/Discoveries
Vitamin*	F. G. Hopkins, Cosimir Funk
Vitamin-A	Mc. Collum
Vitamin-B	Mc. Collum
Vitamin-C	Holst
Vitamin-D	Mc. Collum
Sulpha drugs	Dagmanck (Dogmanck)
Streptomycin	Selman Waksmann
Heart Transplantation	Christian Bernard
Homoeopathy	Hahnemann
Malaria parasite and treatment	Ronald Ross
Diarrhoea and treatment of plague	Kitajato
Sex hormone	Stenach
Open heart surgery	Waltallilehak
Contraceptive pills	Pincus
First test tube baby	Edwards and Stepto

Electrocardiograph	Iwanyaan
Antigen	Karl Landsteiner
RNA	James Watson and Arther Arg
DNA	James Watson and Crick
Insulin	Banting

Funk named it 'Vitamine' (in 1912)

Some Important facts

1. The study of dreams is called Oneirology.
2. The study of the beauty of human is called Kalology.
3. At the time of creation of life there was no oxygen.
4. The strongest part in the body is the enamel of teeth.
5. The sex determination of human depends on male chromosomes not on female chromosomes.
6. The fastest nervous speed is 532 kmph.
7. The internal area of the lungs of human is 93 sq. m. which is forty times of the external area of the body.
8. The bones are as strong as concrete and as hard as granite.
9. Inside the body approximately 150 lakh cells are destroyed every second.
10. The weight of the uterus of the woman who has not given birth to a child is 50 grams and after giving birth to a child the weight becomes 100 grams.
11. The weight of the kidney is approximately 150 grams.
12. In a single inhaling, a normal adult takes 500 ml air inside the body.
13. The capacity of heart to pump the blood is 4.5 liters per minute.
14. The length of the small intestine is approximately 7 meter and its diameter is 2.5 centimeter.
15. The blood circulation inside the body takes approximately 23 seconds.
16. The antibiotic namely, penicillin is obtained from penicillium fungus.
17. Human is the most intelligent hominid of the universe.
18. Albatross is the largest sea bird, whose spread of feather is 10-12 ft.
19. There are approximately 50 lakhs hair in the body of human.
20. In the initial stage of formation of placenta, H.C.G. hormones flow at a large quantity and excreted through urine. At this time, in the testing of urine due to presence of this hormone pregnancy test is carried out.
21. The heart beat of a child is more than that of an adult.
22. A single respiration completes in 5 seconds i.e. 2 seconds of inspiration and 3 seconds of expiration.

23. Everyday blood in the body of the human carries approximately 350 liters of oxygen to the cells of the body. Out of this 97% oxygen is carried by haemoglobin and remaining 3% is circulated by blood plasma.

2. Common Drugs

➪ *Analgesics:* Medicines used to relieve pain

➪ *Antipyretics:* Medicines used to reduce body temperatures.

➪ *Anaesthetics:* Drugs that block the sensory nerves, making a person unconscious. These are used during surgeries so that the patient does not feel any pain.

➪ *Antibiotics:* Medicines used to treat infections caused by microorganisms, such as bacteria etc.

➪ *Antihistamines:* Medicines used to fight the histamine reaction of an allergy, by resisting the action of the histamine.

➪ *Enema:* A fluid which is passed into the rectum for desired bowel movement.

➪ *Lotion:* Medicines used to wash the external body parts in order to cool, soothe or provide antiseptic effect.

➪ *Narcotics:* A drug that is addictive, but reduces pain and changes the mood and behaviour of a person. It also induces sleep.

➪ *Ointment:* A semisolid preparation (usually containing a medicine) applied externally as a remedy or for soothing an irritation.

➪ *Paste:* medicine of soft and sticky consistency; applied externally.

➪ *Sedatives:* Drugs used to induce sleep in a person.

➪ *Suppository:* Medicated mass inserted into the rectum to aid bowel movements.

➪ *Tranquilizers:* Depressant drugs that combat anxiety.

➪ *Vaccines:* Medical substance that provides temporary immunization from contagious diseases.

3. Milestones in Medicine

Invention	Inventor	Year	Country
Stethoscope	Rene Laennec	1819	France
Kidney Machine	Kolf	1944	Netherlands
Sex hormones	Eugen Steinach	1910	Austria
Oral Contraceptive Pills	Gregory Pincus, Rock	1955	USA
Malaria Germs	Laveran	1880	France

First test tube baby	Steptoe and Edwards	1978	Britain
Morphine	Friderich Sertumer	1805	Germany
Cardiac Pacemaker	A.S. Hyman	1932	USA
Cryo- surgery	Henry Swan	1953	USA
Virology	Ivaovski and Bajerick	1892	USSR and Netherlands
Measles Vaccine	Endes	1963	USA
Chloroform as anaesthetic	James Simpson	1847	Britain
Heart Transplant Surgery	Christian Barnard	1967	South Africa
Leprosy Bacillus	Hansen	1873	Norway
Small Pox eradicated	W.H.O. Declaration	1980	UN
Rabies Vaccine	Louis Pasteur	1860	France
Polio Vaccine	Jonas Salk	1954	USA
Synthetic Antigens	Landsteiner	1917	USA
Small Pox Vaccine	Jenner	1776	Britain
Local Anesthesia	Koller	1894	Britain
Blood Bank/Blood Plasma Storage	Drew	1940	USA
Spinal Anesthesia	Bier	1898	Germany
Aspirin	Dreser	1889	Germany
LSD	Hoffman	1943	Switzerland
Chloromycetin	Burkholder	1947	USA
Endocrinology	Bayliss and Starling	1902	Britain
Penicillin	Alexander Fleming	1928	Britain
Open Heart Surgery	Walton Lillehel	1953	USA
Terramycin	Finlay and Others	1950	USA
Vitamin D	Mc Collum	1925	USA
Hypodermic Syringe	Alexander Wood	1853	Britain

Bacteria	Leeuwenhoek	1883	Netherlands
Histology	Marie Bichat	1771-1802	France
Typhus Vaccine	J. Nicolle	1909	France
Vaccination	Edward Jenner	1796	Britain
Cholera T.B. Germs	Robert Koch	1877	Germany
Reserpine	Jal Vakil	1949	India
Gene Therapy on Human	Martin Clive	1980	USA
Vitamin B_1	Minot & Murphy	1936	USA
Embryology	Kari Earnest- Van Baer	1792-1896	Estonia
Physiology	Albrecht Von Haller	1757-66	Switzerland
Serology	Paul Ehrlich	1884-1915	Germany
Polio- Oral vaccine	Albert Sabin	1960	USA
Circulation of blood	William Harvey	1628	Britain
Diphtheria germs	Klebs and Loffler	1883-84	Germany
CAT scanner	Godfrey Hounsfield	1968	Britain
Chemotherapy	Paracelsus	1493-1541	Switzerland
Electro-cardiograph	William Einthoven	1903	Netherlands
Electro-encephalogram	Hand Berger	1929	Germany
Neurology	Franz Joseph Gall	1758-1828	Germany
Rh-factor	Karl Landsteiner	1940	USA
Vitamin K	Doisy Dam	1938	USA
Vitamin C	Froelich Holst	1919	Norway
Blood Transfusion	Jean-Baptiste Denys	1625	France
Recombinant-DNA Paul Berg, S.Cohen, Technology	H.W. Boyer	1972-73	USA
Genes associated Robert	Weinberg with cancer and others	1982	USA

Nuclear magnetic resonance imaging	Raymond Damadian	1971	USA
Vitamin A	Mc Collum and M. Davis	1913	USA
Antitoxins	Behring and Kitasato	1890	Germany & Japan
Biochemistry	Jan Baptista Van Helmont	1648	Belgium
Bacteriology	Ferdinand Cohn	1872	Germany
Positron Emission Tomography	Louis Sokoloff	1978	USA
Meningitis Vaccine	Gardon, et al Cannaught Lab	1987	USA
Thyroxin	Edward Calvin-Kendall	1919	USA
Streptomycin	Selman Waksmann	1944	USA
HIV	Martagnier	1984	France
Pasteurisation	Louis Pasteur	1867	France
MRI	Damadian	1971	USA

4. SI Units or the International System of Units

The International System of Units, abbreviated as the SI Units is the *modern form of the metric system*. It is the world's most widely used system of units, in the field of commerce and science.

The basic SI units are as follows:

SI Base Units		
Base Quantity	**Name**	**Symbol**
Length	Metre	m
Mass	Kilogram	kg
Time	Second	s
Electric Current	Ampere	A
Thermodynamic Temperature	Kelvin	K
Amount of substance	Mole	mol
Luminous Intensity	Candela	cd

The derived SI units are as follows:

Derived Quantity	Name	Symbol
Area	square metre	m^2
Volume	cubic metre	m^3
speed, velocity	metre per second	m/s
Acceleration	metre per second squared	m/s^2
wave number	reciprocal metre	m^{-1}
mass density	kilogram per cubic metre	kg/m^3
specific volume	cubic metre per kilogram	m^3/kg
current density	ampere per square metre	A/m^2
magnetic field strength	ampere per metre	A/m
amount-of-substance concentration	mole per cubic metre	mol/m^3
Luminance	candela per square metre	cd/m^2
mass fraction	kilogram per kilogram, which may be represented by the number, 1	kg/kg $= 1$

For easy understanding, about 22 SI units have been given signs and symbols as follows:

Derived Quantity	Name	Symbol	Expression in terms of other SI units	Expression in terms of SI base units
plane angle	radian (a)	rad	–	$m.m^{-1} = 1$ (b)
solid angle	steradian (a)	sr (c)	–	$m^2.m^{-2} = 1$ (b)
Frequency	hertz	Hz	–	s^{-1}
Force	newton	N	–	$m.kg.s^{-2}$
pressure, stress	pascal	Pa	N/m^2	$m\text{-}1.kg.s^{-2}$
energy, work, quantity of heat	joule	J	N·m	$m^2.kg.s^{-2}$
power, radiant flux	watt	W	J/s	$m^2.kg.s^{-3}$
electric charge, quantity of electricity	coulomb	C	–	s.A

electric potential difference,				
electromotive force	volt	V	W/A	$m^2.kg.s^{-3}.A^{-1}$
Capacitance	farad	F	C/V	$m^{-2}.kg^{-1}.s^4.A^2$
electric resistance	ohm	Ω	V/A	$m^2.kg.s^{-3}.A^{-2}$
electric conductance	siemens	S	A/V	$m^{-2}.kg^{-1}.s^3.A^2$
magnetic flux	weber	Wb	V·s	$m^2.kg.s^{-2}.A^{-1}$
magnetic flux density	tesla	T	Wb/m^2	$kg.s^{-2}.A^{-1}$
Inductance	henry	H	Wb/A	$m^2.kg.s^{-2}.A^{-2}$
Celsius temperature	degree Celsius	°C	–	K
luminous flux	lumen	lm	cd·sr (c)	$m^2.m^{-2}.cd$ = cd
Illuminance	lux	lx	lm/m^2	$m^2.m^{-4}.cd = m^{-2}.cd$
activity (of a radionuclide)	becquerel	Bq	-	s^{-1}
absorbed dose, specific energy (imparted), kerma	gray	Gy	J/kg	$m^2.s^{-2}$
dose equivalent (d)	sievert	Sv	J/kg	$m^2.s^{-2}$
catalytic activity	katal	kat		$s^{-1}.mol$

The following table shows the SI units whose names and symbols include the SI derived units with special names and symbols:

Derived Quantity	Name	Symbol
dynamic viscosity	pascal second	Pa.s
moment of force	newton metre	N.m
surface tension	newton per metre	N/m
angular velocity	radian per second	rad/s
angular acceleration	radian per second squared	rad/s^2

heat flux density, irradiance	watt per square metre	W/m²
heat capacity, entropy	joule per kelvin	J/K
specific heat capacity, specific entropy	joule per kilogram kelvin	J/(kg.K)
specific energy	joule per kilogram	J/kg
thermal conductivity	watt per metre kelvin	W/(m.K)
energy density	joule per cubic metre	J/m³
electric field strength	volt per metre	V/m
electric charge density	coulomb per cubic metre	C/m³
electric flux density	coulomb per square metre	C/m²
Permittivity	farad per metre	F/m
Permeability	henry per metre	H/m
molar energy	joule per mole	J/mol
molar entropy, molar heat capacity	joule per mole kelvin	J/(mol.K)
exposure (x and α rays)	coulomb per kilogram	C/kg
absorbed dose rate	gray per second	Gy/s
radiant intensity	watt per steradian	W/sr
Radiance	watt per square metre steradian	W/(m².sr)
catalytic (activity) concentration	katal per cubic metre	kat/m³

5. Scientific Instruments and their Uses

Instrument	Use
Altimetre	It measures altitudes and is used in aircrafts
Ammetre	It measures strength of electric current (in amperes)
Anemometre	It measures force and velocity of wind
Audiometre	It measures intensity of sound

Audio – Phone	It is used for improving imperfect sense of hearing
Barograph	It is used for continuous recording of atmospheric pressure
Barometre	It measures atmospheric pressure
Binocular	It is used to view distant objects
Bolometre	It measures heat radiation
Calorimetre	It measures quantity of heat
Carburetor	It is used in an internal combustion engine for charging air with petrol vapour
Cardiogram	It traces movements of the heart, recorded on a cardiograph
Chronometre	It determines longitude of a place kept onboard ship
Cinematography	It is an instrument used in cinema making to throw on screen and enlarges the image of a photograph
Crescograph	It measures the growth in plants
Cyclotron	A charged particle accelerator which can accelerate charged particles to high energies
Dynamo	It converts mechanical energy into electrical energy
Dynamometre	It measures electrical power
Electrometre	It measures electricity
Electroscope	It detects presence of an electric charge
Endoscope	It examines internal parts of the body
Eudiometre	Glass tube for measuring volume changes in chemical reactions between gases
Fathometre	It measures the depth of the ocean
Galvanometre	It measures the electric current of low magnitude
Hydrometre	It measures the specific gravity of liquids
Hygrometre	It measures humidity in air
Hydrophone	It measures sound under water
Kymograph	It graphically records physiological movements (Blood pressure and heartbeat)

Lactometre	It determines the purity of milk
Manometre	It measures the pressure of gases
Mariner's Compass	It is an instrument used by the sailors to determine the direction
Microphone	It converts the sound waves into electrical vibrations and to magnify the sound
Microscope	It is used to obtain magnified view of small objects
Odometre	An instrument by which the distance covered by wheeled vehicles is measured
Phonograph	An instrument for producing sound
Photometre	The instrument compares the luminous intensity of the source of light
Periscope	It is used to view objects above the sea level (used in sub-marines)
Potentiometre	It is used for comparing electromotive force of cells
Pyrometre	It measures very high temperature
Radar	It is used for detecting the direction and range of an approaching plane by means of radio microwaves
Rain Gauge	An apparatus for recording rainfall at a particular place
Radiometre	It measures the emission of radiant energy
Refractometre	It measures the refractive index
Saccharimetre	It measures the amount of sugar in the solution
Seismograph	It measures the intensity of earthquake shocks
Salinometre	It determines salinity of a solution
Sextant	This is used by navigators to find the latitude of a place by measuring the elevation above the horizon of the sun or another
Star	
Spectrometre	It is an instrument for measuring the energy distribution of a particular type of radiation
Speedometre	It is an instrument placed in a vehicle to record its speed.

Sphygmoma-nometre	It measures blood pressure
Spherometre	It measures the curvatures of surfaces
Stereoscope	It is used to view two dimensional pictures
Stethoscope	An instrument which is used by the doctors to hear and analyse heart and lung sounds.
Stroboscope	It is used to view rapidly moving objects.
Tachometre	An instrument used in measuring the speeds of aeroplanes and motorboats
Teleprinter	This instrument receives and sends typed messages from one place to another
Telescope	It views distant objects in space
Theodolite	It measures horizontal and vertical angles
Thermometre	This instrument is used for the measurement of temperatures
Thermostat	It regulates the temperature at a particular point
Viscometre	It measures the viscosity of liquids
Voltmetre	It measures the electric potential difference between two points

COMPUTER AND INFORMATION TECHNOLOGY

1. Introduction to Computer

⇨ One of the greatest things that man has ever created is, perhaps, 'the Computer'. The computer is truly an amazing machine. Computer is being used in areas of administration, medicine, education, sports, defence, shops, home, markets and many more. Computer and Information Technology (IT), in recent years, has become an integral part of our life.

⇨ A computer is an electronic machine that helps to process data. It is used to solve problems relating to almost all fields such as education, home, medicine, science and technology, research, designing, publishing, communication etc.

⇨ A computer is an information-processing and information-accessing tool. This means that a computer accepts some information or data from the outside world. It processes it to produce a new information.

⇨ Computer is an electronic device which processes the input informations according to the given set of instructions, called program.

⇨ Blaise Pascal had developed the first mechanical calculator in 1642 AD, which is called 'Pascalene'.

⇨ British scientist Charles Babbage was the first person to conceive an automatic calculator or a computer in 1833. He is called the 'Father of modern computer'.

⇨ The credit of developing first computer program goes to Lady Ada Augusta, a student of Babbage.

⇨ Herman Holorith prepared an electronic tabulating machine in 1880, which was automatically functional with the help of Punch Card. This Punch Card is used in computer even today.

⇨ Howard Ekin developed the first Mechanical Computer 'Mark-I' in 1937.

⇨ J.P. Ekart and John Moschley invented world's first electronic computer 'ENIAC-I' in 1946 and paved the way for first revolution in the field of calculating machine or computer. Electronic Valve or Vaccum Tube was used as a switch in the computer.

⇨ John Van Newman invented EDVAC (Electronic Descrete Variable Computer) in 1951, in which he used Stored Program. The credit of using Binary System in computers also goes to him. Indeed Mr. Newman contributed most in the development of computer and thus gave a right direction to the Computer Revolution (Second Revolution).

2. Generations of Computer

Generation	Period	Main Electronic components	Main Computers
I	1940-52	Electronic Valve Vaccum Tube	EDSAC, EDVAC, UNIVAC
II	1952- 64	Transistor	IBM-700, IBM-1401, IBM-1620, CDC-1604, CDC-3600, ATLAS, ICL-1901
III	1964- 71	Integrated Circuit	IBM-360, IBM-370, NCR-395, CDC-1700, ICL-2903
IV	1971–	Largely Integrated Circuit	APPLE, DCM
V	—	Optical Fibre	

Types of Computer: According to size and capacity the following are types of Computer:

1. **'Micro Computer :** These computers are used by individual, thus also called PC or Personal Computer. These days P.Cs are largely used for domestic and official purposes etc.

2. **Mini Computer :** This type of computer is comparatively larger than that of micro computer. This is 5 to 50 times more powerful than that of a Micro Computer.

3. **Main Frame Computer :** These are large sized computers. By Time Sharing and Multi Tasking techniques many people rather more than 100 people can work at a time on different terminals of this computer.

4. **Super Computer :** These are very powerful computers and have more storage capacity. These are the most expensive and the fastest computers, able to process most complex jobs with a very high speed.

   Super Computers that were developed across the world are:

   (i) Blue Gene manufactured by the IBM Co. of the USA

   (ii) COSMOS manufactured by the Cambridge University of the UK

   (iii) CRAY KIS manufactured by the CRAY K Research Co., USA

   (iv) Deep Blue manufactured by the IBM Co. of the USA

Supercomputers that were developed in India are:

(i)   CHIPP-16 manufactured by C-Dot of Bangalore

(ii) FLO SOLVER manufactured by NAL of Bangalore

(iii) MACH manufactured by IIT of Mumbai

(iv) MULTIMICRO manufactured by IIS of Bangalore

(v) PACE manufactured by the DRDO

(vi) PARAM10000 manufactured by C-DAC of Pune

5. **Quantum Computer :** The development of this type is in final stage. Probably Quantum Computers will be more advanced than that of human brain. In Quantum Computers Q -Bit will be used in lieu of Binary Bits.

Programming Languages of different generations

Generation	Languages
1st Generation (1940-52)	FORTRAN- i
2nd Generation (1952-64)	FORTRAN-ii, ALGOL- 60, COBOL, LISP
3rd Generation (1964-71)	PL/I, ALGOL - W, ALGOL - 68, Pascal, SIMULA- 67, APL, SNOBOL, 4 BASIC, C
4th Generation (1971—)	CLUE, ALFARD, UCLID, Reformed Pascal, MODULA, EDA, ORACLE
5th Generation (For future)	Artificial Intelligence Languages.

Organization of a Computer

⇨ A computer is organized into three basic units:

(i)   Central Processing Unit (CPU)

(ii) Memory Unit (MU) and

(iii) Input/Output Unit

(i) Central Processing Unit (CPU)

The CPU is the part of a computer that performs the main function of information processing. The memory unit stores data. The computer supplies processed information back to the users using special output devices.

⇨ The Central Processing Unit or CPU, is the most important part of the computer. It is called the brain of the computer. It makes all the required calculations and processes data.

⇨ The CPU can be divided into three main components: (a) ALU (b) CU and (c) Registers.

(a) **The Arithmetic and Logic Unit (ALU):** ALU performs all the mathematical and logical operations on the information supplied to the CPU.

(b) **Control Unit (CU):** This unit directs the working of the CPU. It fetches instructions (Programs) from the memory and according to the instructions, controls the flow of data between the ALU and other parts of the computer.

(c) **Registers:** Registers are storage locations that hold instructions or data while the CPU is using them. The registers consist of flip-flops and the registers used by the CPU are the fastest memory elements in the computer. In contrast, the memory unit holds instructions and data before or after the CPU processes these.

Main Attributes of CPU

(a) **Data Width :** It refers to the number of bits of data that can be manipulated within the CPU at one given time.

⇨ The data width of a computer is also called its word size.

⇨ Computers have data widths ranging from 8 to 64 bits.

⇨ A higher data width means the CPU is capable of processing data faster. A CPU with a higher data width is more powerful.

(b) **Address Range:** Address range refers to the amount of memory that can be directly read or written by the CPU.

(c) **Clock Speed:** The speed of CPU is known as Clock Speed. The computer is essentially composed of tiny devices that can be put on or off to indicate 1 or 0.

⇨ At any moment several thousand such devices change their state. To synchronize the change of all these components the CPU uses an internal clock.

⇨ With every tick of this clock all switches that need to change their position do so in perfect harmony.

⇨ The larger the number of ticks per second the faster is the speed of the CPU.

⇨ The ticks per second of the internal clock are measured in megahertz and gigahertz.

⇨ Hertz is a unit of frequency.

⇨ 1 MHz = 1 million ticks per second, 1 GHz = 1000 MHz

⇨ Higher the clock-speed, faster the computer.

(ii) Memory Unit (MU)

The memory unit stores all instructions and data for the CPU. Memory Unit is an important part of the computer system. The storage device of a computer system is known as memory. Memory Unit can receive data, hold it and deliver according to the instructions from the control unit.

⇨ Memory is of two kinds: (a) Primary and (b) Secondary.

(a) Primary Memory

It is often referred to as the working memory or the main memory of a computer system. It is capable of sending and receiving data at a very high speed. It is temporary in nature i.e. Data stored in primary memory are lost when the computer is switched off. So it is also called volatile memory. Example of primary memory is RAM.

⇨ Primary memory is directly accessible to the CPU. It must be able to provide data very quickly.

⇨ The two basic kinds of primary memory are the Random Access Memory (RAM) and the Read Only Memory (ROM).

⇨ The RAM is a read/write memory.

⇨ The CPU can change the contents of the RAM at any time. In addition, RAM is volatile.

⇨ The RAM capacity greatly influences the computing ability of the computer. Capacity is usually measured in kilobytes and megabytes.

⇨ The ROM can not be altered.

⇨ Informations is stored on the ROM at the time of its manufacture. The information might be in the form of crucial instructions that govern the working of the computer.

⇨ The ROM is non-volatile and retains its information even after the power is turned off.

⇨ The PROM (Programmable Read Only Memory), however, has the option of being programmed, i.e. the manufacturer of the computer may choose to load a program designed by his company into this PROM, and then the computer would use this PROM like any other ROM.

(b) Secondary Memory

It is used to store data for a long term. It operates at a much slower rate than primary memory. Secondary memory is permanent in nature, so it is also called non-volatile. It is also cheaper than primary memory. Examples of secondary memory are floppy disks, hard disks, magnetic tapes etc.

⇨ Primary memory is fast but expensive. To reduce storage costs, computers also use secondary memory.

⇨ It is not directly accessible to the CPU. Information is moved from the secondary memory to the primary memory first and then to the CPU.

⇨ Common examples of secondary memory are floppy diskettes, hard (fixed) discs and magnetic tapes.

⇨ A floppy diskette is a plastic disk coated with magnetic material.

- Special devices known as disk drives are capable of reading from and writing to floppies using special magnetic head'.
- Any piece of information stored on a floppy diskette can be directly accessed.
- Magnetic tapes are long plastic tapes coated with magnetic material.
- Magnetic tapes can store far larger amounts of data than the floppy diskette. But a problem with magnetic tapes is that information cannot be accessed directly as in the case of floppy diskettes.
- The third type of medium, called fixed or hard disks, are more or less similar to the floppy diskette. But one hard disk drive contains several discs of a hard material.
- Another popular storage medium is the compact disk (CD). Unlike the media described above, CDs are an 'optical medium.
- An optical medium is one where the properties of light are used for the medium to perform its basic functions.
- Conventional CDs are made of a special kind of plastic.
- The CD is read using a laser beam.
- Secondary memory is much slower, but it is non-volatile and can be used to store information for long periods of time.

(iii) Input/Output

- There has to be a physical channel that permits users to supply informations to the computer.
- Devices that permit users to supply information to the computer are called 'input' devices.
- Input unit enables us to enter (or Input) data into a computer. The common input devices are keyboard and mouse.
- Similarly, a physical channel that permits a computer to convey the processed information to the outside world. Devices that permit such a function are called 'output' devices.
- Output unit enables the computer to show us the result and the information that we want. The common output devices are monitor, printer and speakers.
- Input and output devices are indispensable, but are not a part of the CPU. They are also called peripheral devices, suggesting that they lie on the periphery of the CPU.
- These devices are also called an interface, because they translate information for man and machine.
- The most popular input device used in contemporary computers is the keyboard.

- Another way to input information into a computer is to use an Optical Mark Reader (OMR). Optical Mark Readers are capable of reading specially prepared forms. These forms have a provision for black marks to be made using a pen or a pencil in a specific position.
- Most competitive examinations that deal with a large number of students usually use this system.
- Banks use another input device called a Magnetic Ink Character Reader (MICR).
- Special numbers are written on bank cheques using magnetic ink and in a particular style to write different numbers. The MICR passes over the words or characters, examines the shape of the magnetic field created by the character, and is thus able to recognize it.
- Bar codes are often imprinted on products in merchandise stores. A bar code consists of several parallel vertical lines of different thickness that represent the binary digits.
- The bits form a code that can be used to identify the object on which the bar code is imprinted. A bar code reader is used to read the bar codes by detecting the bars by using light.
- The bar code can represent information like the price of the product or its date of expiry etc.
- Menu-driven programs, where the user sees the host of on-screen choices, sometimes use another input devices called the mouse.
- The mouse is a pointing device. It can be gripped in the palm of the hand and moved over a horizontal surface. The motion of the mouse can be monitored by the computer in different ways.
- The movement is measured and transmitted to the computer. This generates a corresponding movement of an on-screen marker called a cursor from one option to another.
- To select an option, the user presses one of the mouse's buttons.
- Another input device is a digital camera. A digital camera has a circuit that is sensitive to light.
- The two most common devices are the Visual Display Unit (VDU) and the printer.
- A Visual Display Unit (VDU) uses a cathode ray tube to display informations.
- To represent any character, VDU illuminates a particular pattern of these dots. These dots are also known as pixels, a short form for picture-elements.

- Printers print characters on paper or other similar medium.
- Printers come in three popular versions : dot matrix printers, ink-jet printers and laser printers.
- Dot matrix printers print characters in the form of combinations of very tiny dots. The printing head aligns its 'pins' to match a particular pattern of dots.
- Ink-jet printers spray jets of ink on to the paper to print any character. The characters are absolutely smooth as ink is sprayed in a continuous flow.
- Laser printer uses a laser beam to actually burn the characters on to the paper.
- We need to issue the computer a detailed sequence of instructions that it needs to follow to operate upon any data. Such a sequence is called a program.
- A program may directly be written to the RAM or may be stored in some form of secondary memory.
- It may be transferred from the secondary memory to the RAM as and when required.
- Execution of a program means that data is moved around in the CPU according to a well-detailed sequence by the programme.
- Computer programs are written using special languages called programming languages.
- There are several programming languages. Each language has its own grammar called its syntax.

3. Computer Networking and Internet

A computer network, or simply a network, is a collection of computers and other hardware interconnected by communication channels that allow sharing of resources and information.Where at least one process in one device is able to send/receive data to/from at least one process residing in a remote device, then the two devices are said to be in a network. A network is a group of devices connected to each other. Networks may be classified into a wide variety of characteristics, such as the medium used to transport the data, communications protocol used, scale, topology, benefit, and organisational scope.

Communication protocols define the rules and data formats for ex-changing information in a computer network, and provide the basis for network programming. Well-known communication protocols include two Ethernet, a hardware and link layer standard that is ubiquitous in local area networks, and the Internet protocol suite, which defines a set of protocols for inter-networking, i.e. for data communication between multiple networks, as well as host-to-host data transfer, and application-specific data transmission formats.

Computer networking is sometimes considered a sub-discipline of electrical engineering, telecommunications, computer science, information technology or computer engineering, since it relies upon the theoretical and practical application of these disciplines.

Internet

The Internet is a global system of interconnected governmental, academic, corporate, public and private computer networks. It is based on the networking technologies of the Internet Protocol Suite. It is the successor of the Advanced Research Projects Agency Network (ARPANET) developed by DARPA of the United States Department of Defense. The Internet is also the communications backbone underlying the World Wide Web (WWW).

Participants in the Internet use a diverse array of methods of several hundred documented, and often standardized, protocols compatible with the Internet Protocol Suite and an addressing system (IP addresses) administered by the Internet Assigned Numbers Authority and address registries. Service providers and large enterprises exchange information about the reachability of their address spaces through the Border Gateway Protocol (BGP), forming a redundant worldwide mesh of transmission paths.

Most traditional communications media including telephone, music, film, and television are being reshaped or redefined by the Internet, giving birth to new services such as Voice over Internet Protocol (VoIP) and Internet Protocol Television (IPTV). Newspaper, book and other print publishing are adapting to Web site technology, or are reshaped into blogging and web feeds. The Internet has enabled and accelerated new forms of human interactions through instant messaging, Internet forums, and social networking. Online shopping has boomed both for major retail outlets and small artisans and traders. Business-to-business and financial services on the Internet affect supply chains across entire industries.

The origins of the Internet reach back to research of the 1960s, commissioned by the United States government to build robust, fault-tolerant, and distributed computer networks. The funding of a new U.S. backbone by the National Science Foundation in the 1980s, as well as private funding for other commercial backbones, led to worldwide participation in the development of new networking technologies, and the merger of many networks. The commercialization of what was by the 1990s an international network resulted in its popularization and incorporation into virtually every aspect of modern human life. As of June 2012, more than 2.4 billion people — over a third of the world's human population — have used the services of the Internet.

The Internet has no centralized governance in either technological implementation or policies for access and usage; each constituent network sets its own standards. Only the overreaching definitions of the two principal name spaces in the Internet, the Internet Protocol address space and the Domain Name System, are directed by a maintainer organisation, the Internet Corporation for Assigned Names and Numbers (ICANN). The technical underpinning and standardization of the core protocols (IPv4 and IPv6) is an activity of the Internet Engineering Task Force (IETF), a non-profit organisation of loosely affiliated international participants that anyone may associate with by contributing technical expertise.

4. Computer Terminology

Computer terminology helps us to understand the technical terms of the world of computers. The following are some important terms used in computer operation:

⇨ **active program or window** – The application or window at the front (foreground) on the monitor.

⇨ **alert** (alert box) – a message that appears on screen, usually to tell you something went wrong.

⇨ **alias** – an icon that points to a file, folder or application (System 7).

⇨ **apple menu** – on the left side of the screen header. System 6 is equal to desk accessories, System 7 is equal to up to 50 items.

⇨ **application** – a program in which you do your work.

⇨ **application menu** - on the right side of the screen header. Lists running applications.

⇨ **ASCII** (pronounced ask-key) – American Standard Code for Information Interchange. A commonly used data format for exchanging information between computers or programs.

⇨ **bit** – the smallest piece of information used by the computer. Derived from "binary digit". In computer language, either a one (1) or a zero (0).

⇨ **backup** – a copy of a file or disk you make for archiving the purposes.

⇨ **boot** – to start up a computer.

⇨ **bug** – a programming error that causes a program to behave in an unexpected way.

⇨ **bus** – an electronic pathway through which data is transmitted between components in a computer.

⇨ **byte** – a piece of computer information made up of eight bits.

⇨ **card** – a printed circuit board that adds some feature to a computer.

⇨ **cartridge drive** – a storage device, like a hard drive, in which the medium is a cartridge that can be removed.

⇨ **CD-ROM** – an acronym for Compact Disc Read-Only Memory.

⇨ **command** – the act of giving an instruction to your MAC either by menu choice or keystroke.

⇨ **command (apple) key** – a modifier key, the Command key used in conjunction with another keystroke to active some function on the MAC.

⇨ **compiler** – a program the converts programming code into a form that can be used by a computer.

⇨ **compression** – a technique that reduces the size of a saved file by elimination or encoding redundancies (i.e., JPEG, MPEG, LZW, etc.)

⇨ **control key** – seldom used modifier key on the MAC.

⇨ **control panel** – a program that allows you to change settings in a program or change the way a MAC looks and/or behaves.

⇨ **daisy chaining** – the act of stringing devices together in a series (such as SCSI).

⇨ **database** – an electronic list of information that can be sorted and/or searched.

⇨ **data** – (the plural of datum) information processed by a computer.

⇨ **defragment** – (also optimize) to concatenate fragments of data into contiguous blocks in memory or on a hard drive.

⇨ **disk** – a spinning platter made of magnetic or optically etched material on which data can be stored.

⇨ **disk drive** – the machinery that writes the data from a disk and/or writes data to a disk.

⇨ **disk window** – the window that displays the contents or directory of a disk.

⇨ **DPI** — acronym for Dots Per Inch — a gauge of visual clarity on the printed page or on the computer screen.

⇨ **Ethernet** – a protocol for fast communication and file transfer across a network.

⇨ **expansion slot** – a connector inside the computer which allows one to plug in a printed circuit board that provides new or enhanced features.

- **file** – the generic word for an application, document, control panel or other computer data.
- **finder** – The cornerstone or home-base application in the MAC environment. The finder regulates the file management functions of the MAC (copying, renaming, deleting...)
- **footprint** – The surface area of a desk or table which is occupied by a piece of equipment.
- **fragmentation** – The breaking up of a file into many separate locations in memory or on a disk.
- **gig** – a gigabyte = 1024 megabytes.
- **K** – kilobyte.
- **keyboard shortcut** – a combination of keystrokes that performs some function otherwise found in a pulldown menu.
- **kilobyte** – 1024 bytes.
- **landscape** – in printing from a computer, to print sideways on the page.
- **Measurements** (summary) :
  - a bit = one binary digit (1 or 0) 'bit' is derived from the contraction b'it (binary digit) -> 8 bits = one byte
  - 1024 bytes = one kilobyte
  - K = kilobyte
  - Kb = kilobit
  - MB = megabyte
  - Mb = megabit
  - MB/s = megabytes per second
  - Mb/s = megabits per second
  - bps = bits per second i.e., 155 Mb/s = 19.38 MB/s
- **One megabyte** — 1024 kilobytes.
- **multi finder** – a component of System 6 that allows the *Mac* to multi task.
- **multi-tasking** – running more than one application in memory at the same time.
- **nanosecond** – one billionth of a second. (or, the time between the theatrical release of a Dudley Moore film and the moment it begins to play on airplanes).
- **native mode** – using the computers original operating system; most commonly used when talking about the PowerPC can run software written for either the 80x0 systems, or the PowerPCs RISC code.

⇨ **partition** – a subdivision of a hard drives surface that is defined and used as a separate drive.

⇨ **PCI** – acronym for Peripheral Component Interchange - the newer, faster bus achitecture.

⇨ **point** – (1/72″) 12 points = one pica in printing.

⇨ **pop-up menu** – a menu that does not appear at the top of the screen in the menu bar. (may pop up or down)

⇨ **RISC** – acronym for Reduced Instruction Set Computing; the smaller set of commands used by the PowerPC and Power *Mac*.

⇨ **ROM** – acronym for Read Only Memory; memory that can only be read from and not written to.

⇨ **root directory** – the main hard drive window.

⇨ **SCSI** – acronym for Small Computer System Interface.

⇨ **SCSI address** – a number between zero and seven that must be unique to each device in a SCSI chain. Fast and Wide SCSI devices will allow up to 15 SCSI IDs (hexidecimal); however, the length restriction (3 metres) is such that it is virtually impossible to link 15 devices together.

⇨ **SCSI port** – a 25 pin connector on the back of a MAC (native SCSI port); used to connect SCSI devices to the CPU. Some SCSI cards (like the ATTO) have a 68 pin connector.

⇨ **SCSI terminator** – a device placed at the end of a SCSI chain to complete the circuit. (some SCSI devices are self-terminating, or have active termination and do not require this plug).

⇨ **serial port** – a port that allows data to be transmitted in a series (one after the other), such as the printer and modem ports on a MAC.

⇨ **server** – a central computer dedicated to sending and receiving data from other computers (on a network).

⇨ **spreadsheet** – a program designed to look like an electronic ledger.

⇨ **start up disk** – the disk containing system software and is designated to be used to start the computer.

⇨ **surge suppressor** – a power strip that has circuits designed to reduce the effects of surge in electrical power. (not the same as a UPS)

⇨ **System file** – a file in the System folder that allows your MAC to start and run.

⇨ **System folder** – an all-important folder that contains at least the System file and the Finder.

⇨ **32 bit addressing** – a feature that allows the MAC to recognize and use more than 8 MB of memory.

- ➪ **Uninterruptible Power Source** (UPS) – a constantly charging battery pack which powers the computer. A UPS should have enough charge to power your computer for several minutes in the event of a total power failure, giving you time to save your work and safely shut down.
- ➪ **vaporware** – "software" advertised, and sometimes sold, that does not yet exist in a releasable for.
- ➪ **virtual memory** – using part of your hard drive as though it were "RAM".
- ➪ **WORM** – acronym for Write Once-Read Many; an optical disk that can only be written to once (like a CD-ROM).
- ➪ **zoom box** – a small square in the upper right corner of a window which, when clicked, will expand the window to fill the whole screen.

6. Abbreviations Associated with Computer

CDAC	Centre for Development of Advanced Parallel Computing
CDOT	Centre for Development of Telematrics
HTTP	HyperText Transfer Protocol
ROM	Read Only Memory
RAM	Random Access Memory
BEGOS	Basic Input-Output System
MODEM	Modulation-Demodulation
CAD	Computer Aided Design
PSTN	Public Switched Telephone Network
PSPDN	Pocket Switched Public Data Network
RAB MN	Remote Area Business Message Network
LAN	Local Area Network
WAN	Wide Area Network
MAN	Metropolitan Area Network
CDMA	Code Division Multiple Access
GAIS	Gateway Internet Access Service
E-Mail	Electronic Mail
CD	Compact Disc
LDU	Liquid Display Unit
CPU	Central Processing Unit
CAM	Computer Aided Manufacturing

CATScan	Computerised Axial Tomography Scan
COBOL	Common Business Oriented Language
COMAL	Common Algorithmic Language
DOS	Disc Operating System
DTS	Desk Top System
DTP	Desk Top Publishing
E-Commerce	Electronic Commerce
ENIAC	Electronic Numerical Integrator And Calculator
FAX	Fascimile Automated Xerox
FLOPS	Floating Operations Per Second
FORTRAN	Formula Translation
HLL	High Level Language
HTML	Hyper Text Markup Language
IBM	International Business Machine
IC	Integrated Circuit
ISH	International Super Highway
LSP	List Processing
LLL	Low Level Language
MICR	Magnetic Ink Character Recognition/Reader
MIPS	Millions of Instructions Per Second
MOPS	Millions of Operations Per Second
MPU	Micro Processor Unit
NICNET	National Informatics Centre Network
OMR	Optical Mark Reader/Recognition
PC-DOT	Personal Computer Disk Operation System
PROM	Programmable Read Only Memory
SNOBOL	String Oriented Symbolic Language
UPS	Uninterruptable Power Supply
VDU	Visual Display Unit
VLSI	Very Large Scale Integrated
WWW	World Wide Web

www.ingramcontent.com/pod-product-compliance
Lightning Source LLC
Chambersburg PA
CBHW072232270326
41930CB00010B/2101